SECOND EDITION

Mastering Concept-Based Teaching

A Guide for Nurse Educators

JEAN FORET GIDDENS, PhD, RN, FAAN, ANEF
Dean and Professor
School of Nursing
Virginia Commonwealth University
Richmond, Virginia

LINDA CAPUTI, EdD, MSN, CNE, ANEF
President
Linda Caputi, Inc.
Nursing Education Consultant
Professor Emerita
College of DuPage
Glen Ellyn, Illinois

BETH RODGERS, PhD, RN, FAAN
Professor
School of Nursing
Virginia Commonwealth University
Richmond, Virginia

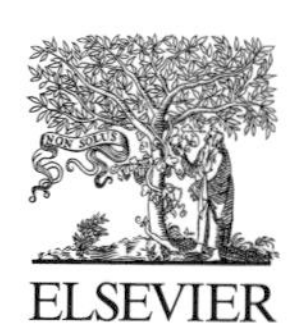

ELSEVIER

MASTERING CONCEPT-BASED TEACHING, A GUIDE FOR NURSE EDUCATORS, SECOND EDITION
ISBN: 978-0-323-55460-2

Notices

Library of Congress Control Number: 2018962581

Library of Congress
US Programs, Law, and Literature Division
Cataloging in Publication Program
101 Independence Avenue, S.E.
Washington, DC 20540-4283

Content Strategist: Lee Henderson
Content Development Manager: Ellen Wurm-Cutter
Content Development Specialist: Laura Klein
Publishing Services Manager: Shereen Jameel
Project Manager: Radhika Sivalingam
Design Direction: Patrick Ferguson

Printed in the United States of America

Last digit is the print number: 9 8 7 6 5 4 3 2 1

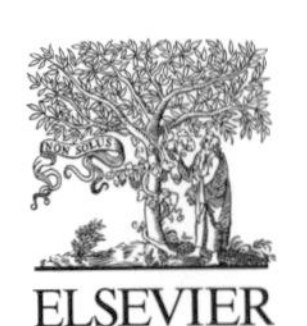

3251 Riverport Lane
St. Louis, Missouri 63043

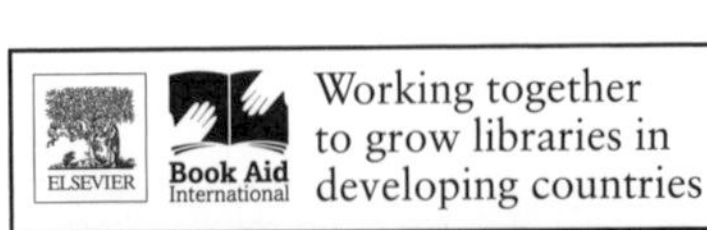

Mastering Concept-Based Teaching

A Guide for Nurse Educators

ABOUT THE AUTHORS

Jean Giddens
Dr. Giddens earned a Bachelor of Science in Nursing from the University of Kansas, a Master of Science of Nursing from the University of Texas at El Paso, and a PhD in Education and Human Resource Studies from Colorado State University. Dr. Giddens has more than 25 years' experience in associate-degree, baccalaureate-degree, and graduate-degree nursing programs in New Mexico, Texas, Colorado, and Virginia. She is an expert in concept-based curriculum and evaluation, as well as innovative strategies for teaching and learning. Dr. Giddens serves as an education consultant to nursing programs throughout the country and is the author of multiple journal articles, electronic media, and nursing textbooks, including *Concepts for Nursing Practice.*

Linda Caputi
Dr. Caputi earned an MSN from Loyola University, Chicago, and an EdD from Northern Illinois University. She is a Certified Nurse Educator and a fellow in the National League for Nursing's Academy of Nursing Education. Dr. Caputi is Professor Emeritus, College of DuPage. She has won six awards for teaching excellence from Sigma Theta Tau and has been included for 3 years in *Who's Who Among America's Teachers*. She is the author or editor of five books, chapter contributor for six books, and has published many journal articles, all on nursing education. Dr. Caputi is President of Linda Caputi, Inc., a nursing education consulting company, and she has worked with hundreds of nursing programs related to revising curriculum, transforming clinical education, and numerous other nursing education topics.

Beth Rodgers
Dr. Rodgers earned a Bachelor of Science degree in Nursing from Georgia State University and an MSN and PhD in Nursing from the University of Virginia. She has devoted more than 28 years to nursing education at the undergraduate and graduate levels and to research to expand knowledge about the experiences of people living with chronic conditions. She is recognized widely for her expertise in nursing as a discipline and the development of nursing knowledge, and Dr. Rodgers is frequently sought as a consultant in nursing epistemology, as well as concept and theory development in doctoral education in nursing. She is the author or editor of two popular textbooks on knowledge and concept development, along with an extensive array of book chapters and journal articles.

PREFACE

The education reform movement over the past 2 decades has been propelled by an expansion in what we know related to human learning. Advances in brain research related to the process of thinking and learning have had a significant influence on the practice of teaching. Research has shown that learning is influenced by the ability to make connections between information and that such connections form knowledge structures that facilitate the application of information to multiple situations. This process is at the heart of the *conceptual approach*. Thus, the science of learning has led to the rise of the conceptual approach in primary and secondary education, as well as higher education. In recent years, significant interest in the conceptual approach has grown in nursing education. This increased interest parallels the education discipline and is seen as a way to manage excessive curriculum content through information management, to engage students, to develop the thinking skills of nursing students, and to produce highly skilled nursing graduates who can manage patients in an increasingly complex health care system.

The conceptual approach represents the incorporation of concepts, exemplars, concept-based curriculum, concept-based instruction, and conceptual learning into the practice of nurse educators. For most faculty, the conceptual approach represents a considerable change in the way the curriculum is structured and taught. It requires a collective reframing of the education process among faculty and students. Although there is significant interest in adopting the conceptual approach in nursing programs, many faculty groups have not had adequate exposure to this approach or clear guidance and therefore lack the expertise or understanding. They may have teaching expertise but just not in conceptual teaching, which is needed for optimal success.

This book was written specifically as a resource for the conceptual approach in nursing education. Targeted users of this book include nursing faculty in undergraduate or graduate nursing programs and graduate nursing students who are preparing for a career in academia. This book does not attempt to replicate the many excellent resources that exist related to general education on faculty roles, teaching strategies, and curriculum development. However, this book does present these topics within the context of the conceptual approach. It is also not expected that an individual will read this book sequentially from cover to cover—so each chapter stands alone and is beneficial in relation to the desired topic area.

- Chapter 1 focuses on the conceptual approach as a general overview. It is an excellent starting point for faculty who want a broad "30,000-foot" view of the conceptual approach and the various elements.
- Chapters 2 and 3 provide a deep look into concepts and understanding what is meant by concept analysis; these chapters are presented from a theoretical lens and are intended to deepen the understanding of concepts; this understanding is foundational to the conceptual approach.
- Chapter 4 provides a discussion about how to develop a concept-based curriculum. Although this process mirrors any other curriculum development process, concepts are used as the infrastructure for the curriculum, and this chapter explains how.
- Chapter 5 offers readers a look into what is now known about how the human brain learns and how the use of concepts enhances learning.
- Chapter 6 presents a discussion of conceptual teaching for the classroom setting and how this differs from traditional content-focused instruction. Furthermore, the reader is provided examples of specific teaching strategies that result in conceptual learning.
- Chapter 7 presents a discussion of conceptual teaching in the clinical setting and how examples-focused learning activities focused on concepts.

- Chapter 8 presents an overview of evaluation strategies that faculty can use to determine achievement of student learning—again with a specific emphasis on conceptual learning, as well as strategies for program evaluation for schools with a concept-based curriculum.
- Chapter 9 provides the reader with an overview of the nursing literature as it relates to the conceptual approach and suggestions for developing expertise in the conceptual approach.

Important to note, the nine chapters in this book are closely interrelated to one another—in other words, some overlap is unavoidable. For example, part of the development and implementation of a concept-based curriculum (Chapter 4) includes the development of teaching strategies (Chapters 6 and 7) and the curriculum evaluation plan (Chapter 8). As another example, the development of effective teaching strategies (Chapters 6 and 7) requires the foundational understanding of concepts (Chapters 2 and 3) and an understanding of human learning with concepts (Chapter 5).

This book represents the collaborative efforts of three experienced nurse educators with the intent of harnessing their wide and varied expertise into a useful resource for our faculty colleagues who are courageous enough to embark on the conceptual approach journey. We hope this book will serve you well along the way!

Jean Giddens

Linda Caputi

Beth Rodgers

ACKNOWLEDGMENTS

It has been my honor and privilege to work with my two colleagues, Linda Caputi and Beth Rodgers, on this book. Their extraordinary expertise has led to a deepening of my own conceptual understandings. I also extend my gratitude and appreciation to our colleagues at Elsevier, Lee Henderson, a long-time colleague and advocate, and Laura Klein, who helped us stay on schedule and navigated our work through production. Lastly, I extend my sincere gratitude to our nursing faculty colleagues for moving our profession forward. May the torch burn long and bright!

JFG

TABLE OF CONTENTS

CHAPTER 1

The Conceptual Approach—Background and Benefits

Jean Giddens

If you have been a nurse educator anytime during the past decade, you have likely noticed significant movement toward the conceptual approach as a basis for curriculum design and teaching. Perhaps you heard about this approach at a conference or from a colleague or read about it in a journal article. Perhaps one or more faculty members from your nursing program have discussed the possibility of adopting a concept-based curriculum as part of a curriculum redesign. Perhaps you are part of a faculty group that is actively developing or implementing a concept-based curriculum. Regardless of how or where you have heard about it, the conceptual approach has been a recent and important trend in nursing education, and its use has been growing exponentially.

You may be wondering what all the buzz is about. Is the conceptual approach merely a gimmicky trend that will pass, or is it part of a transformation of nursing education that is desperately needed? Indeed, educators should be careful not to jump on every bandwagon that comes along. In many cases, education innovations gain immediate interest but are quickly abandoned when implementation proves challenging and or when outcomes fall short of expectations. Most nurse educators have very full workloads and must make the best use of their time. Thus, with regard to any trend, educators are encouraged to consider what is reasonable and not reasonable and what is supported by education science.

A conceptual approach in nursing education may be adopted for many reasons. Among the most important reasons are to manage excessive curriculum content through information management, engage students, develop the thinking skills of nursing students, and produce nursing graduates who are highly skilled in the management of patients in a health care system that is increasingly complex. Successful adoption and implementation of the conceptual approach requires nurse educators to transform the learning environment from the traditional teacher-focused delivery of information to a student-centered environment in which students are actively engaged in the learning process. Carrieri-Kohlman, Lindsey, and West (2003) describe the conceptual approach as "a process that deliberately attempts to examine the nature and substance of nursing from a conceptual perspective" (p. 1). For most nursing programs, the conceptual approach represents a cultural shift in the way faculty and students perceive their roles in the teaching-learning process. The purpose of this chapter is to provide historic background regarding concept-based approaches in education and nursing, describe what is meant by the *conceptual approach*, and present benefits of the conceptual approach for contemporary nursing education.

Background

Many nurse educators might be surprised to learn that the conceptual approach is not a new trend but rather has been borrowed from another discipline and adapted to nursing. Two interesting historical perspectives are associated with the conceptual approach, one from the education discipline and the other from nursing.

THE EARLY YEARS

In the education discipline, curriculum was historically approached by discrete areas and topical organizers for content. The emphasis for curriculum development was on the selection and organization of content around topical organizers (such as math, social studies, sciences, etc.) with educational objectives primarily targeting basic knowledge acquisition. Student learning focused on memorization of facts and the practice of discrete skills. As an example, a traditional approach to learning the mathematic skill of multiplication involves memorizing columns of multiplication equations with answers. Other examples include memorizing rules of grammar or memorizing all 50 state capitals. This is not to say that rote learning does not have benefits; the ability to recall basic facts provides a necessary foundation for conceptual learning. However, rote learning and memorization do not develop active thinking necessary for higher level problem solving.

As early as the 1950s, Hilda Taba, a visionary educator from San Francisco, proposed the notion of concepts as opposed to topics as content organizers. She emphasized developing the capability of discriminating essential from nonessential information. In her work, concepts are referred to as high-level abstractions, and she proposed inductive strategies for concept formation. Taba postulated that a person's understanding of a concept expands when challenged with increasingly complex examples representing the concept (Taba, 1966). At that time, critics of her work raised concerns about the abstract nature of concepts. It was recognized that unless concepts were clearly defined, they were challenging for faculty to teach in a clear and efficient way.

During this same general period in nursing, many grand theories were emerging, such as those proposed by Abdellah, Johnson, Rogers, Orem, King, Roy (Marriner-Tomy & Alligood, 2006). The era of grand theories was a reflection of nursing as a maturing discipline. Nursing grand theories represent the organization, arrangement, or framework of key concepts and principles that describe the profession. These theories provided a mechanism for the nursing profession to clearly establish itself as a unique and separate health care discipline. Defining professional identity is important work for any profession on its continuum of ongoing development. Subsequently, in the 1970s and 1980s, the design of nursing curricula based on a grand theory became common practice. Because concepts associated with the chosen theory were often used as the foundation for the curriculum, many of these curricula were referred to as "concept based." For example, Orem's Self-Care Framework (Orem, 1971) was widely used as a basis for curriculum development. Orem's theory included the following concepts:

- Self-care
- Self-care agency
- Therapeutic self-care demand
- Self-care deficit
- Nursing agency
- Nursing system

These concepts serve as the building blocks of Orem's theory and are very useful in that context. However, use of these as foundational concepts for a nursing curriculum was problematic for many nursing programs when faculty did not clearly understand the concepts and did not know how to teach conceptually or how to link specific content to the concepts. Although nursing faculty in some schools were successful with this type of curriculum design, many educators struggled to translate abstract theoretical concepts to practical application, particularly when teaching novice learners. Interestingly, some of these same issues were experienced within the education discipline.

EDUCATION REFORM

It was not until the 1990s that significant education reform propelled the idea of different models of curricula and different approaches to teaching. In a study of science and mathematics education, authors described curricula in the United States as "an inch deep and a mile wide" (Schmidt, McKnight, & Raizen, 1997). It became increasingly obvious to educators that the massive content covered in education was limiting true cognitive development (Erikson, 2002). At the same time, increased attention was being directed at research into human learning. In the late 1990s, the National Research Council conducted a study that led to the publication of *How People Learn* (Bransford, Brown, & Cocking, 2000), which provided a synthesis on the science of learning. Bransford and colleagues noted a convergence of evidence across many disciplines, with significant implications for education. Advances in brain research related to the process of thinking and learning have influenced teaching, curriculum design, instructional assessment, and learning environments. As a result, an emphasis on linking brain research (and the research of learning) to teaching practice has increased over the past decade. One of the themes noted from the research is the notion that learning is influenced by students' ability to make connections between information. Structural changes in the brain occur through a process called *neuroplasticity*—in other words, neurons build connections in response to learning. These neurological connections form knowledge structures that allow learners to apply information and knowledge effectively to multiple situations—including new situations. This process is at the heart of the conceptual approach. Thus the science of learning has influenced the rise of a concept-based curriculum as an alternative to the traditional curriculum models in primary and secondary education (Erikson, 2002, 2008).

THE CONCEPTUAL APPROACH MOVEMENT IN NURSING EDUCATION

Although nursing has been slower to embrace changes in teaching and curriculum design, many nurse educators have taken cues from the education discipline and are becoming increasingly aware of the science supporting new models for teaching and learning, and they are reexamining concept-based approaches. The current conceptual approach movement in nursing began in the mid-2000s. Unlike concept-based curricula of the past (which were largely based on a single grand theory), contemporary concept-based models in nursing education feature common concepts that have emerged from nursing science as the profession has matured. The expansion of concepts presented in the context of nursing is reflected in the nursing literature, particularly during the last 25 years. Thus the primary distinctions in present-day concept-based models compared with those of the past are that (1) more concepts have been defined and formally developed, (2) the concepts are less abstract (and easier for faculty and students to understand), and (3) advances in the science of teaching and learning are applied.

MISCONCEPTIONS AND CLARIFICATIONS

Misconception: The conceptual approach is a new idea from the nursing discipline that has emerged over the last decade and is spreading to other disciplines.

Clarification: The conceptual approach was proposed in the 1950s with origins in primary and secondary education. Today it is being applied in many disciplines and levels of education.

The Conceptual Approach

Because many ideas and terms are used to describe the conceptual approach trend in nursing education, clarification is important as a starting point. The term *conceptual approach* in education is broad and represents the incorporation of the following separate but interrelated elements: concepts,

BOX 1.1 ■ Elements of the Conceptual Approach

- **Concept:** An organizing idea or mental image composed of attributes.
- **Exemplar:** A specific topic or an example represented by the concept.
- **Concept-Based Curriculum:** A curriculum that is designed by organizing content around key concepts.
- **Concept-Based Instruction:** An instructional process featuring student-centered learning activities that focuses on concepts and the application of information to concepts.
- **Conceptual Learning:** A process by which learners develop high-level thinking skills and the ability to apply facts in the context of related concepts.

exemplars, concept-based curriculum, concept-based instruction, and conceptual learning (Box 1.1). These elements are briefly described here and will be expanded on in various chapters throughout this text.

ELEMENTS OF THE CONCEPTUAL APPROACH

Concepts

Central to the conceptual approach are concepts. A concept is an organizing idea or mental construct represented by common attributes. Rodgers describes concepts as "an abstraction that is expressed in some form" (1989, p. 332). Key terms to focus on in the two concept descriptions above are *mental construct* and *abstraction*. Important to note is that a concept is not a physical object – you can't directly see, touch, taste, or smell a concept. Concepts are ideas or the organization of thoughts formed in the mind. Concepts are often represented by physical things. For example, the concept of *Fruit* is a mental construct we all share. Physical objects that represent the concept of fruit include apples, oranges, and bananas. Put another way, you can't eat the concept of *Fruit*, but a bowl of strawberries (which represents the concept of *Fruit*) is delicious! However, it is not always so simple. Some concepts do not have any physical objects to represent them. For example, the concept of *Beauty* is more abstract than the concept of *Fruit* because of the variability in the interpretation of beauty. *Beauty* can be associated with objects (such as flowers or jewelry) or less tangible things such as landscapes, personality, or a spiritual experience. In other words, for some concepts, the exemplars are abstractions in themselves.

In the conceptual approach, concepts form the infrastructure of a concept-based curriculum and are the key elements associated with concept-based instruction and conceptual learning. Concepts represent the key ideas that are used to organize knowledge, facts, skills, and competencies across multiple situations and contexts. Concepts function as hubs for transferable knowledge.

Any given discipline, including nursing, contains an endless number of concepts that range from the very broad (known as *macroconcepts*) to the narrow (known as *microconcepts*). Several concepts can link to each macroconcept, and several microconcepts can link to each concept (Figure 1.1). The designation of macroconcept, concept, and microconcept is context specific. In other words, what is considered a concept for undergraduate nursing education might be considered a macroconcept for an expert in a given area; likewise, what is considered an advanced or microconcept for an undergraduate student may be considered a basic concept to an expert. For example, *Ethics* is widely considered an appropriate concept for nursing education. As a way to frame the scope of *Ethics* as a concept, four ethical principles—autonomy, beneficence, nonmaleficence, and justice—might be used. However, an advanced scholar and expert in this area might consider *Ethics* as a macro concept, with four primary concepts: *Autonomy, Beneficence, Nonmaleficence*, and *Justice*. Thus a crucial task of educators who adopt the conceptual approach is to not only identify and clearly address key concepts to be used, but also ensure that the appropriate level of concept is selected for the learner.

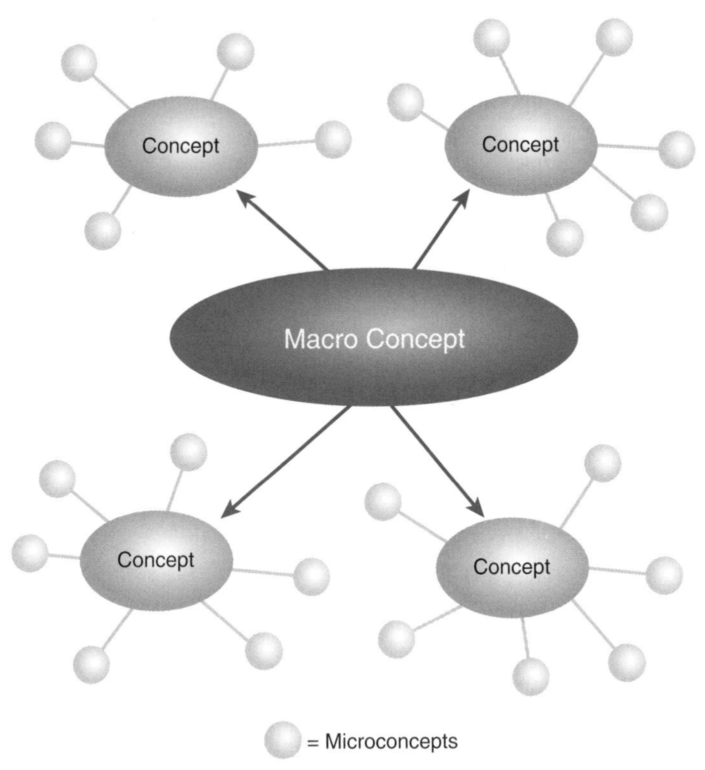

Fig. 1.1 Relationship between macroconcepts, concepts, and microconcepts. Macroconcepts are broad and abstract with multiple associated concepts. Microconcepts are narrow, specific, and tend to be associated with specialty practice/knowledge.

Not only should concepts be selected on the basis of relevancy to the discipline and the program of study, but they also should be organized logically within the curriculum and be used consistently by faculty for maximum benefit to the learner. Achieving such consistency among faculty requires a solid understanding (and agreement) of how the concepts are to be used in the curriculum across courses, how to present the concepts in a useful way to students, and how to link essential content knowledge to the concepts for in-depth understanding. Additionally, faculty must help students recognize the relationships among the key concepts, because in most clinical situations several concepts are involved (which are referred to as *interrelated concepts*). For example, Figure 1.2 shows the concept *Health Promotion* and several key interrelated concepts. In this example, three different concept categories are represented: *Health and Illness* (at the right), *Professional Nursing* (at bottom, left), and *Patient Attribute* (top). Each of these interrelated concepts not only link to health promotion but also link to each other (as illustrated by the arrows). Interrelated concept diagrams help visualize the interrelationships and illustrate the complexity of concepts. Concepts are discussed in greater detail in Chapters 2 and 3.

Exemplars

Exemplars represent specific examples of a topic. For a concept-based curriculum, the exemplars are the most important examples, topics, or content related to a concept. Typically there are many exemplars for any given concept, and exemplars usually connect to multiple concepts. In other words, a concept is not represented by only one exemplar, and an exemplar can represent many

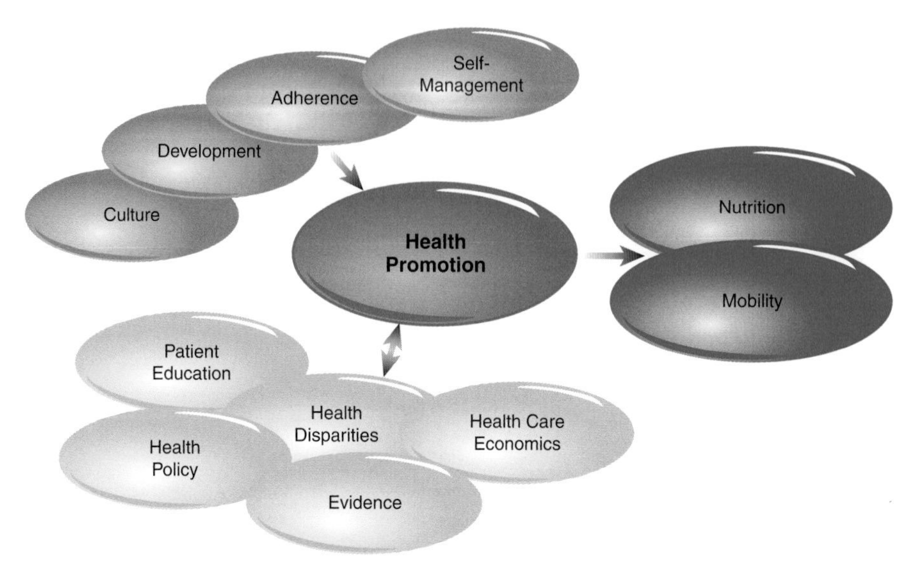

Fig. 1.2 Health promotion and interrelated concepts. Interrelationships among health care recipient concepts, health and illness concepts, and professional nursing concepts. (From Giddens J. *Concepts for Nursing Practice*. 2nd ed. St. Louis, MO: Elsevier; 2017.)

very different concepts. For example, returning to the previous example of *Fruit* as a concept, many types of *Fruit* could be used as exemplars including apples and strawberries. However, apples and strawberries could also be used as exemplars of the concept of red.

In nursing, exemplars are an essential component of the conceptual approach because they represent essential content knowledge. It is worth noting that facts remain an important component of learning. Facts represent specific information embedded within exemplars; thus students build conceptual understandings based on an accurate knowledgebase. The complex interrelationship between facts/topics, exemplars, concepts, and macroconcepts is at the heart of gaining conceptual understandings. Figure 1.3 illustrates this complex relationship. Exemplars provide specific context and help students grasp a deep understanding of the concept. In nursing, exemplars can be health-related conditions experienced by patients (such as asthma, a hip fracture, or an allergic reaction); situations experienced by patients and families in the context of health (such as death and dying, caregiver roles, developmental delays, and bullying); or situations experienced by nurses in the context of professional nursing practice (such as informed consent, delegation of care, medication teaching, and quality improvement projects).

One of the fundamental tasks of nurse educators who are adopting the conceptual approach is to identify the exemplars to be used for each concept. Faculty members often feel compelled to include multiple exemplars for each concept (often content from their own specialty or content they have traditionally taught) because of their belief that the content is critical and that students must know it. However, one of the benefits of the conceptual approach is information management, and thus the exemplars should be limited to those most representative or important in helping students attain a grasp of the concept. The learning emphasis should be on the development of cognitive connections back to the concept—in other words, the student should not only learn about the exemplar, but how it relates back to one or more concepts. Because exemplars typically link to multiple concepts, faculty should incorporate exemplars in the curriculum plan in such a way that repetitious use of a particular exemplar is avoided. For example, pneumonia could be used effectively as an exemplar for the concepts of gas exchange, infection, acid-base

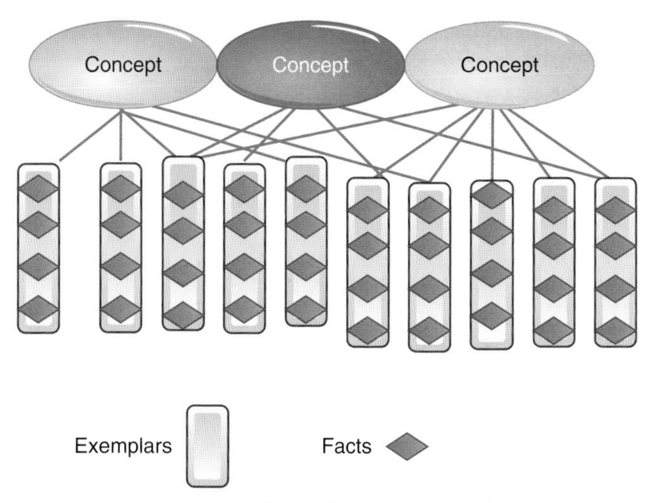

Fig. 1.3 Concepts, exemplars, and facts. The relationship between facts, exemplars, and concepts is complex.

balance, or fatigue. However, it would be unwise to use pneumonia four times within the curriculum as an exemplar, especially considering the many other key content areas that students need to learn. Faculty must help students make purposeful cognitive connections from the exemplar to the primary concept and to other key interrelated concepts. This is a necessary step to avoid information overload.

A Concept-Based Curriculum

A third element of the conceptual approach is a concept-based curriculum, in which concepts serve as "foundational organizers" that provide an infrastructure to the curriculum. A concept-based curriculum represents a major paradigm shift for nursing because it moves away from an emphasis on content and toward an emphasis on concepts and conceptual learning (Giddens & Brady, 2007). Featured concepts within the courses serve as cornerstones for concept-based instruction and conceptual learning (Giddens et al., 2008). Lynn Erikson, a leading expert in concept-based curriculum and instruction, describes the differences between content-focused and concept-focused curricula as "the difference between memorizing facts related to the American Revolution and developing and sharing ideas related to the concepts of freedom and independence as a result of studying the American Revolution" (Erikson, 2002, p. 50).

When a concept-based curriculum is designed, several key decisions must be made. As with any curriculum, faculty should first determine desired program learning outcomes. After this initial step, concept categories or an organizing framework should be developed, and concepts should be selected. Each concept should be developed so that faculty members gain a shared understanding about what the concept means and what it represents. Exemplars that will be linked to each concept also must be chosen. Exemplar selection should be based on the best examples of the concept or the most common situations represented. Next, decisions regarding the type of courses and the arrangement of concepts within courses must be made, followed by the actual development of each course, and the plan for teaching within the course. Curriculum development also includes a general plan for evaluation to ensure that students attain program learning outcomes, such as demonstrating competencies. Implementation issues include faculty development, student orientation, and maintaining the curriculum integrity. These key decisions and issues are summarized in Box 1.2 and are described further in Chapter 4

BOX 1.2 ■ Key Steps and Decisions When Designing a Concept-Based Curriculum

1. Review mission, vision, and values of institution/school.
2. Develop program outcomes.
3. Develop an organizing framework for concepts.
4. Select and develop featured curriculum concepts.
5. Identify exemplars for each concept.
6. Organize concepts and exemplars into courses/course development.
7. Develop a program evaluation plan.

Concept-Based Instruction

A fourth element associated with the conceptual approach is concept-based instruction. This instructional process is characterized by student-centered learning activities that focus on *target concepts* (meaning the featured concept for a unit of study) and the application of key exemplars to concepts. It is worth mentioning again that the focus of instruction is on both the concept (such as a concept overview) *and* the specific exemplars linked to that concept.

How does one actually teach a concept? A typical starting point is the concept overview (or concept presentation). A concept overview includes the concept definition, scope or categories of the concept, concept attributes, assessment, process and consequences and nursing management. Faculty incorporate important facts and information as foundational to learning the concept. As an example, students must understand learning domains (cognitive domain, psychomotor domain, and affective domain), as well as educational approaches, before they can grasp the concept of patient education. The use of facts in foundational information is absolutely necessary as part of the conceptual learning process because facts support conceptual learning; conceptual learning leads to conceptual understanding, which supports the students' ability to make generalizations.

The concept overview is followed by the application of exemplars to deepen the students' understanding of the concept. A deep understanding of the concept leads to the ability of the student to form generalizations and relationships between concepts. It is also important to note that there is not a single or specific instructional strategy for conceptual teaching. Concept-based instruction incorporates a variety of teaching strategies and learning experiences that require higher levels of thinking from faculty and students (Erikson, 2008). Ideally, students are placed in learning groups and work through cases, situations, questions, or problems posed by the instructor as opposed to faculty-centered lectures on concepts. Chapters 6 and 7 are devoted to concept-based instructional strategies that support conceptual learning.

Conceptual Learning

Conceptual learning is an active process that engages students and results in synergistic thinking. Timpson and Bendel-Simso (1996) described conceptual learning as a process through which students learn to organize information into logical mental structures and become increasingly skilled at thinking. During the learning process, students link factual information and exemplars to concepts. Students gain an understanding of the concept through a concept overview and then by actively applying information learned to the concept—and making cognitive links and generalizations to other information. The desired learning outcome is an in-depth understanding of the concept and the ability to transfer ideas to other situations through these cognitive connections. Faculty should be aware, however, that learners must have accurate baseline understandings of information on which to build. Students with inaccurate understanding of information will build on these, leading to further inaccuracies as learning occurs. For this reason, there is value in reviewing and clarifying previously learned information. In nursing, learning experiences ideally should be placed in the context of a clinical situation and should be purposeful; in other words, learners should clearly recognize the benefit of what they are learning as it pertains to the practice of nursing. Engagement in learning is enhanced when students perceive learning as purposeful and they can see a direct application to their area of study (Ambrose, Bridges, DiPietro, Lovette, & Norman, 2010; Bransford, 2000; Sousa, 2010). Conceptual learning is presented in greater depth in Chapter 5.

MISCONCEPTIONS AND CLARIFICATIONS

Misconception: The conceptual approach is a new idea from the nursing discipline that has emerged over the last decade and is spreading to other disciplines.

Clarification: The conceptual approach was proposed in the 1950s with origins in primary and secondary education. Today it is being applied in many disciplines and levels of education.

COHESIVENESS OF THE ELEMENTS

The Greek philosopher Aristotle is credited with coining the phrase, "The whole is greater than the sum of its parts." This phrase captures the significance of the conceptual approach as a cohesive, comprehensive plan as opposed to a loose collection of one or more elements. The conceptual approach requires a purposeful and planned process whereby concepts influence curriculum design, teaching, and learning. This distinction is important because the incorporation of all five elements (see Box 1.1) is necessary for a successful concept-based educational platform. Although each element stands on its own, a powerful synergistic effect occurs when all the elements are meaningfully incorporated into an education plan. Successful adoption of the conceptual approach in nursing requires a commitment among faculty to follow a concept-based curriculum and to learn how to teach conceptually through carefully designed instructional strategies. Students should be actively engaged in the learning process by applying content in purposeful ways and by learning to make cognitive connections to concepts. The end goal is for learners to gain a deep understanding of the concept and acquire the ability to transfer ideas to other concepts and contexts. This outcome represents the higher-level thinking skills necessary for sound clinical judgment in patient care settings. Consider the following two scenarios:

Scenario 1

Faculty members of an undergraduate nursing program work very hard to develop a concept-based curriculum. As part of this process, they write learning outcomes, identify key nursing concepts from the literature, agree on exemplars, and develop courses around the concepts. Although some of the faculty members attempt to incorporate more student-centered learning activities in their approach to teaching, the majority continue to use the traditional lecture format and focus primarily on exemplars with little to no linkage to the concepts. Additionally, several faculty members become concerned about the loss of what they consider to be "essential information" and add content back into their courses.

Scenario 2

Janice teaches a nursing skills lab in a nursing program that has not undergone a significant curriculum revision in 15 years. After attending a conference presentation on conceptual teaching and learning, Janice decides to adopt a concept-based instructional approach for her course. She identifies key concepts for each unit and uses student-centered teaching strategies to help students link their course content and skills to concepts within her course. Students enrolled in Janice's course find that her teaching strategies are different from those of other faculty. Although most students like the way the course is taught, some students become angry because Janice does not just give them the information they need for the course examinations.

In the first scenario, faculty undoubtedly spent significant time and energy to redesign the curriculum and are proud to have a concept-based curriculum. However, two primary elements associated with the conceptual approach are missing: a lack of commitment among faculty to adopt concept-based instruction, and a lost opportunity for students to benefit from a conceptual learning experience. The fact that some faculty members elected to add additional content into their courses further undermines the benefit of adopting a concept-based curriculum.

In the second scenario, Janice is motivated to change her teaching methods. By incorporating student-centered learning activities into her teaching plan, Janice is becoming increasingly comfortable with and skilled in concept-based instruction. She is also providing an engaging learning environment that is enjoyed by most students in her course. However, because no mechanism is in place for students to encounter the concepts in other courses within the curriculum, the experience occurs in isolation with limited effect.

Although the specific situation in each scenario is different, both scenarios are similar in that one or more elements of the conceptual approach were adopted. However, long-term benefits are unlikely to be achieved because one or more key elements of the conceptual approach were not incorporated. Does this mean that complete consensus must be achieved among faculty before they adopt the conceptual approach for their nursing programs? Absolutely not! Gaining complete consensus among any faculty group is unrealistic because of the very nature of academe. A diversity of perspectives, opinions, and values is expected in all organizations. However, for successful adoption of the conceptual approach, critical mass is needed; in other words, adequate support must exist among faculty who teach in the program, and support from the administrative leadership is also necessary.

Benefits of the Conceptual Approach

We are in the midst of widespread change regarding what is known about human learning. What started as a trickle effect has become a force that is changing the landscape of education. The education of students in all disciplines—including nursing—is being dramatically influenced by these events. The conceptual approach links well with this change and offers multiple known benefits, which include addressing content saturation and information management and preparing nurses to successfully practice in complex health care environments by developing conceptual thinking skills that lead to good clinical judgment and collaboration.

ADDRESSING CONTENT SATURATION

Most educators agree that one of their greatest challenges is having sufficient time to teach all the curriculum content. Although concerns about excessive curriculum content have appeared in the nursing literature for more than 30 years, increased attention has been directed at this issue during the past decade (Deane & Asselin, 2015; Diekelmann, 2002; Forbes & Hickey, 2009; Giddens & Brady, 2007; Hendricks & Wangerin, 2017; Ironside, 2004; National League for Nursing, 2003). Excessive content can be partly attributable to what has been known as the "information age." The exponential generation of new information makes it impossible not only to teach everything that is known in a given discipline but also to keep up with advances and changes in what was previously known. It has been estimated that as much as 50% of the information learned in a 4-year degree program changes within 2 years after graduation. This issue is exacerbated by the traditional "instructor-centric" approach to teaching. Faculty who subscribe to this perspective believe they must "cover" all the content, and the common belief is that students cannot be expected to know anything unless it has been specifically taught in a course. This expectation is quite a burden for any faculty member to carry! With this perspective, classroom time typically becomes little more than information delivery sessions as opposed to learning sessions. Excessive curriculum content has also coincided with the increased size of nursing textbooks (because of the increased generation of nursing knowledge). Many faculty feel obligated to cover large amounts of the information found in textbooks rather than encouraging students to use these books as a learning resource and reference. It is easy to see how the cycle perpetuates the problem. The conceptual approach alleviates the issue of content saturation by limiting the number of concepts and exemplars used and by emphasizing students' ability to make linkages to content to which they are exposed, even if it has not been through formal learning activities within the curriculum. The adage "less is more" applies here, not only in terms of the delivery of content, but more importantly, in the result of better learning.

INFORMATION MANAGEMENT

A curriculum focused on content generally emphasizes student memorization of facts (as they are known at that point in time) and does little to prepare students to manage the large volume of changing information they will encounter not only as students but also throughout their career. Information management refers to the ability to *locate, analyze, interpret*, and *apply* new information to specific situations. Because it is impossible for any health care professional to know all the information needed to care for all patients, health care professionals must be highly skilled in information management as a basis for evidence-based care. Nursing education must shift from information delivery to the creation of learning environments in which students are required to locate, analyze, interpret, and apply information as part of learning within classroom, laboratory, and clinical environments. These elements are also foundational to conceptual learning. The conceptual approach fosters students' development of information management by learning to link new and emerging information to concept-structures. These elements are described in the following sections, and an example is provided in Box 1.3.

Locate Information

Health care professionals must know how and where to efficiently locate accurate information on which to base their practice. More specifically, this ability means knowing appropriate and reliable sources (for example, practice, policy, or procedure guidelines and evidence-based practice findings) and having the skill to access these sources (such as through the Internet, Intranet, or a resource manual).

BOX 1.3 ■ Exemplar: Information Management in Practice

Terrin, a nurse working in an inpatient unit, has an order to administer a new pharmacologic agent with which he is unfamiliar. He is told that the agent has only been available for use for 6 months. Terrin logs onto the hospital Intranet website **(locate)** to review the drug information and administration guidelines. Terrin carefully reads the drug information and notices that there are two indications for using the agent; he also notes that the administration guidelines are dependent on many variables, including intended use, age, weight, and underlying medical conditions **(analyze)**. Based on the information presented, Terrin gains an understanding regarding the specific context for which the agent was ordered **(interpret)**. He uses this information to administer the agent correctly and to monitor the patient for potential adverse effects **(apply)**.

Analyze Information

Analysis of information requires a critical examination of information elements to determine the relationship of the parts or to discover meaning. New information and the supporting evidence are often complex, requiring careful consideration of all elements. Health care professionals must be able to gain an accurate understanding of new information through analysis of the information that is available.

Interpret Information

The process of information analysis should lead to the ability of the health care professional to draw meaning from the information. One aspect of the process is to analyze the information, but a key component is the ability to translate the information into understandable terms or context. The process of interpretation means gaining an understanding of the meaning or significance of the information. This process means gaining an understanding of how the information fits with the context of care within the clinical environment.

Apply Information

The evidence-based practice movement ultimately is about applying the latest evidence or information to one's practice. Application of information refers to the process of putting newly learned or discovered information to use. It is assumed that the newly discovered/learned information comes from a reliable source. In the context of health care, the information must be applied correctly to provide evidence-based care.

STUDENT LEARNING AND ENGAGEMENT

Another significant benefit of the conceptual approach is the emphasis on student learning as opposed to the instruction provided by faculty. By and large, the emphasis in education has been on what the instructor does; this notion is captured very well by Bellack, who noted that "...nursing education continues to be 'teaching heavy' and 'learning light'" (Bellack, 2008, p. 439). With the conceptual approach, learning occurs when students develop skills in building cognitive connections to previous learning as opposed to learning facts. The end result is that learners become more effective and efficient thinkers and problem solvers.

COLLABORATION

Effective, coordinated health care delivery depends on collaboration among health care professionals. Teamwork and Collaboration, one of the six core competencies from Quality & Safety Education for Nurses, emphasizes the need for nurses to be skilled collaborators, not only with other nurses but also with persons from other disciplines (QSEN, 2013). Teams and Teamwork is also a core competency identified by the Interprofessional Education Collaborative Expert Panel (IPEC, 2011). Thus there is little doubt that graduates of nursing programs need a strong foundation in collaboration. Collaborative learning is at the heart of the conceptual approach. Historically, higher education has rewarded individual achievement, and this perspective is reinforced in a traditional classroom, where students take in information and are tested on the content. The conceptual approach requires students to learn in groups, and thus collaborative learning in school translates well to collaboration in clinical practice. If nurse educators are sincere in setting expectations that nursing graduates "play well with others," then collaborative learning must occur as a part of the education process from the first to last semesters.

In addition to facilitating collaborative learning, the conceptual approach also provides a platform to design interprofessional learning activities, events, and courses. Most concepts

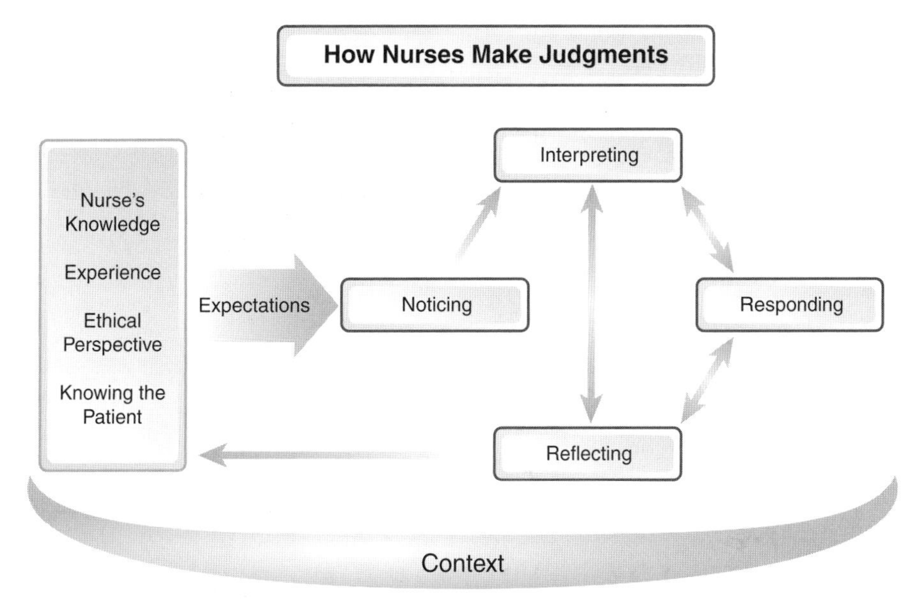

Fig. 1.4 Tanner's Model of Clinical Judgment. (Adapted from Tanner CA. Thinking like a nurse: a research-based model of clinical judgment in nursing. *Journal of Nursing Education.* 2002;45(60):204–211.)

found in a nursing curriculum actually apply to all health care disciplines. For example, students enrolled in medicine, nursing, pharmacy, dentistry, or physical therapy all must learn about concepts such as *Culture, Ethics, Health Promotion, Informatics, Quality, Safety, Infection,* and *Gas Exchange.* Despite the fact that many of these concepts have universal application, each discipline plays a unique role in the provision of health care as it relates to the concepts. The conceptual approach provides a unique opportunity for the development of a robust core interprofessional curriculum featuring collaborative learning and team-based care across disciplines.

FROM CONCEPTUAL THINKING TO CLINICAL JUDGMENT

Nursing graduates must develop skill in clinical reasoning and clinical judgment for success in an increasingly complex health care environment. The linear approach to learning in traditional content-focused curricula does little to facilitate skills needed by nurses in the complex health care system. Tanner's model of clinical judgment (Tanner, 2006) illustrates that a nurse's response to a clinical situation is influenced by his or her previous experiences with regard to a situation, noticing when patterns are inconsistent with a given situation (i.e., taking into consideration the context of the situation), and correctly interpreting and clarifying information (Figure 1.4). The development of conceptual thinking skills facilitates clinical reasoning because of the cognitive connections to concepts made by students when encountering new information. Having an in-depth understanding of a concept provides the necessary platform for students and practicing nurses.

Summary

As the health care environment becomes increasingly complex, nursing programs need to respond by preparing graduates to manage information effectively, provide patient-centered care that is evidence based, and work well within teams. This requires a transformation of nursing education curricula and teaching practices from an instructor-centered and content-focused paradigm to the conceptual approach. This chapter introduces the conceptual approach, reinforcing the notion that five key elements—concepts, exemplars, concept-based curriculum, concept-based instruction, and conceptual learning—must be in place for optimal success (see Box 1.1). Benefits of the conceptual approach include addressing content saturation, information management, enhanced student learning and engagement, collaboration, and supporting the development of clinical judgment. In the chapters that follow, key elements and processes are presented in greater detail to enhance understanding and application in teaching practice.

References

Ambrose SA, Bridges MW, DiPietro M, Lovette MC, Norman MK. *How Learning Works. 7 Research-Based Principles for Smart Teaching*. San Francisco, CA: Jossey-Bass; 2010.

Bellack J. Letting go of the rock. *J Nurs Educ*. 2008;47(10):439–440.

Bransford JD, Brown AL, Cocking RR. *How People Learn: Brain, Mind, Experience, and School*. Washington, DC: National Academy Press; 2000.

Carrieri-Kohlman V, Lindsey AM, West CM. *Pathophysiological Phenomena in Nursing: Human Response to Illness*. 3rd ed. Philadelphia, PA: Saunders; 2003.

Deane W, Asselin M. Transitioning to concept-based teaching: a discussion of strategies and the use of Bridge's change model. *J Nurs Educ Pract*. 2015;5(10):52–59.

Diekelmann N. "Too much content...." Epistemologies' grasp and nursing education. *J Nurs Educ*. 2002;41(11):469–470.

Erikson L. *Concept-Based Curriculum and Instruction*. Thousand Oaks, CA: Corwin Press; 2002.

Erikson L. *Stirring the Head, Heart, and Soul. Redefining Curriculum, Instruction, and Concept-Based Learning*. Thousand Oaks, CA: Corwin Press; 2008.

Forbes MO, Hickey MT. Curriculum reform in baccalaureate nursing education: review of the literature. *Int J Nurs Educ Schol*. 2009;6(1):Article 27.

Giddens J, Brady D. Rescuing nursing education from content saturation: the case for a concept-based curriculum. *J Nurs Educ*. 2007;46(2):65–69.

Giddens J, Brady D, Brown P, Wright M, Smith D, Harris J. A new curriculum for a new era of nursing education. *Nurs Educ Perspect*. 2008;29(4):200–204.

Hendricks SM, Wangerin V. Concept-based curriculum: changing attitudes and overcoming barriers. *Nurs Educ*. 2017;42(3):138–142.

Interprofessional Education Collaborative Expert Panel. Core Competencies for Interprofessional Collaborative Practice: Report of an Expert Panel. Washington, DC: Interprofessional Education Collaborative; 2011.

Ironside PM. "Covering content" and teaching thinking: deconstructing the additive curriculum. *J Nurs Educ*. 2004;43(1):5–12.

Marriner-Tomy A, Alligood MR. *Nursing Theorists and Their Work*. St. Louis, MO: Elsevier; 2006.

National League for Nursing. Position statement: Innovation in nursing education: A call to reform. http://www.nln.org/docs/default-source/about/archived-position-statements/innovation-in-nursing-education-a-call-to-reform-pdf.pdf?sfvrsn=4; 2003.

Orem D, Nursing. *Concepts of Practice*. Columbus, OH: McGraw-Hill; 1971.

Quality & Safety Education for Nurses Institute. *Competencies*. n.d. http://qsen.org/competencies/

Rodgers B. Concepts, analysis, and the development of nursing knowledge: the evolutionary cycle. *J Adv Nurs*. 1989;14:330–335.

Schmidt WH, McKnight CC, Raizen S. *A Splintered Vision: an Investigation of U.S. Science and Mathematics Education. U.S. National Research Center for the Third International Mathematics and Science Study (TIMSS)*. Dordrecht, Netherlands: Kluwer Academic Publishers; 1997.

Sousa DA. *Mind, Brain, and Education. Neuroscience Implications for the Classroom*. Bloomington, IN: Solution Tree Press; 2010.

Taba H. *Teaching Strategies and Cognitive Functioning in Elementary School Children. Cooperative Research Project*. Washington, DC: Office of Education, U.S. Department of Health, Education, and Welfare; 1966.

Tanner CA. Thinking like a nurse: a research-based model of clinical judgment in nursing. *J Nurs Educ.* 2006;45(6):204–211.

Timpson WM, Bendel-Simso P. *Concepts and Choices for Teaching: Meeting the Challenges in Higher Education.* Madison, WI: Magna Publications; 1996.

CHAPTER 2

Concepts in the Discipline of Nursing

Beth Rodgers

Concept-based curricula and a concept-focused approach to teaching are not new phenomena, as noted elsewhere in this book. However, the conceptual approach to teaching is likely to be new for many nurse educators who are more accustomed to focusing on content in the form of "facts" rather than on broader ideas or concepts. An irony is inherent in the idea that a conceptual approach may be unique, however, because human beings work with concepts all the time. In fact, most of what nurses do is based on having a good grasp of the concepts critical to nursing practice. Learning is, to a great extent, a process of concept acquisition, and knowledge involves the formation, clarification, and application of concepts. A concept-based curriculum and a conceptual approach to teaching both require that the conceptual foundation for nursing be at the forefront of teaching and learning. In traditional approaches to teaching, facts and examples receive most of the attention, with thinking about those facts and examples occurring on a more abstract level; in the conceptual approach, thinking takes center stage. For this approach to be successful, faculty who work with students for conceptual learning must have a thorough understanding of concepts, including what they are, how they are formed, how they are used in nursing, how they make up the discipline of nursing, and what functions they serve with regard to knowledge overall. Attempts to implement a conceptual approach to teaching and learning cannot be successful if the faculty do not have a basic grasp of concepts in general.

An Overview of Concepts in Nursing Education

As noted previously, a concept-based approach to teaching helps put a focus on knowing rather than doing. Nurses are strikingly adept at answering questions about what nursing is with an emphasis on what they are able to do or what tasks they perform in the course of their work. When an individual nurse is asked, "What is it like to be a nurse?" a common response often is, "Well, I work in (setting) and do...." The response may even include a reference to the ubiquitous "caring," a gerund that sometimes implies action and tasks. It is important, however, that nurses be able to understand and talk about the knowledge that underlies their actions. Nursing cannot advance as a discipline without recognition of the vast knowledge that nurses hold and that is essential to their actions. A focus on concepts and conceptual learning makes it possible to take the knowledge that the nurse possesses and look at it in the abstract, outside of an immediate application, initially, thus helping to recognize that there is thought and cognitive power in the concept. That thought or knowledge then can be applied to nursing situations that include patient care or other health-related foci. A nurse with a strong conceptual grasp of the discipline, instead of describing tasks, would talk about the creation of empathic relationships with care recipients, whether they be individuals, families, or communities. A nurse who works with persons who have chronic heart disease, for example, would not answer a question about nursing by saying, "I explain their medications, teach them about pacing their activities, and tell them how to monitor their weight." Instead, the nurse can describe work with this population by discussing concepts such as *Mobility*, *Gas Exchange*, and *Self-Management* to help the patient adjust his or her activities to achieve a level of independence and quality of life that is consistent with individual life goals and physiological capacities. The nurse also could relay that he or she has a strong grasp of the illness trajectory and the threats to identity that often accompany chronic illness and, rather than focusing primarily on monitoring for medication adherence and physiological stability or deterioration, works with an understanding of what it is like to live with a chronic condition to help the patient maintain dignity and self-worth. The nurse also would understand the importance of social support in such a situation and work with the patient to develop appropriate strategies to achieve reasonable goals in the situation. Such a description would be quite a change from how a nurse otherwise might describe this type of work, perhaps saying merely, "I work with people who have heart disease."

This approach sometimes is confused with "holism," an important aspect of nursing and one of the characteristics that differentiates it from other disciplines. A holistic focus, however, is not the same as a conceptual focus. Holism refers to how the nurse uses the concepts to approach a patient, family, or community health situation. Holism involves the use of multiple concepts to address the many factors and challenges that are present in any encounter. Holism thus provides a perspective or framework for ensuring that multiple concepts are addressed in the situation as appropriate. A conceptual focus emphasizes the concepts and knowledge that are used to create that holistic approach. A focus on concepts thus is a focus on knowledge first, rather than action. Clearly, knowledge should precede action, and such a focus in the acquisition of cognitive content enables more widespread application than a focus on specific tasks or activities would allow.

A good example of one of the differences in concept-based learning is the concept of *Asepsis*. In a skills-oriented course, the nursing student will learn how to insert an indwelling urinary catheter and all of the appropriate steps in that process. The student also will learn about isolation technique, handwashing, and numerous other physical skills. If the student has a strong grasp of the concept of *Asepsis*, however, he or she can apply that cognitive content across this variety of physical actions. Without the concept of *Asepsis*, the student is in a position of memorizing the steps of each procedure as if they were unrelated. A solid understanding of a concept enables the student (or anyone who grasps the concept) to identify similarities across situations and transfer knowledge from one context to the next. The understanding of *Asepsis* that accompanies having a good grasp of the concept enables the application of knowledge in a variety of situations.

This example using the concept of *Asepsis* reveals one valuable feature of concepts: They are important organizational elements, providing a way of clustering knowledge that enables someone with a strong grasp of a concept to move from one situation to another with some knowledge that helps that person interpret the new situation. Nurses cannot approach every encounter as a completely unique situation, nor can they manage each interaction as if it were an isolated case study. It is necessary to have some way of grasping information and organizing it so it is available for application across varied encounters. Concepts serve that purpose, making it possible to carry knowledge from one situation to another (Figure 2.1). In applying the concepts, it also becomes clear when the concepts need to be refined or improved to be of greater use. In the case of more abstract concepts, such as *Dignity*, *Quality of Life*, or *Autonomy*, there is a theoretical power that is evident and important to nursing practice. Knowledge about such important aspects of human existence cannot be obtained by learning how to name something or by pointing to an object and saying, "That is *Dignity*." No physical objects correspond to such concepts; consequently, it is not possible even to discuss such things without at least a beginning grasp of the concept. Concepts therefore serve an important role in learning and in terms of nursing knowledge in that they are very powerful theoretical clusters of knowledge.

This emphasis on knowledge and the ability to learn and carry information from one situation to the next are key aspects of a conceptual approach to teaching and learning. To enact such an approach, it is necessary to have a thorough understanding of what is meant by the term

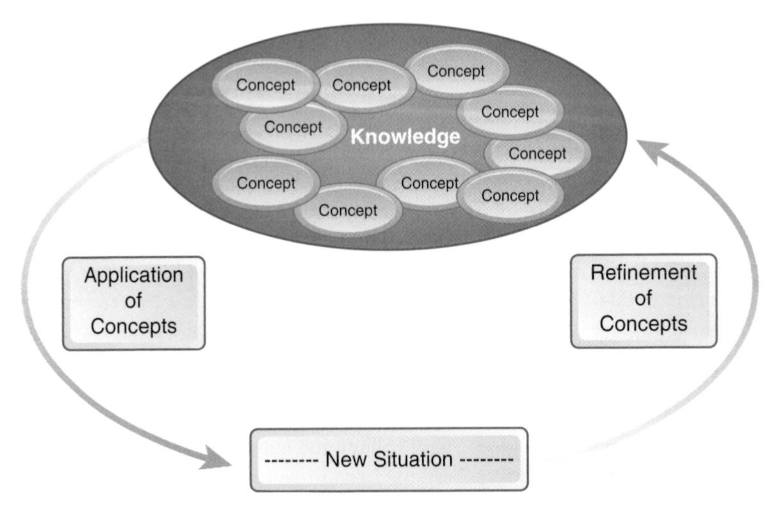

Fig. 2.1 Concepts are used to apply knowledge from one situation to another, resulting in concept refinement. Concepts are used to apply knowledge from one situation to another, resulting in concept refinement.

"concept." In other words, the educator, as well as the student, must have a meaningful concept of what a *concept* is. It is also important to understand how concepts are communicated and shared. Without some way to discuss concepts and share ideas, a conceptual approach to teaching and a concept-based curriculum would not be possible. Language and experience also need to be considered because they are important components of an understanding of concepts.

In nursing, concepts have been identified as important elements of knowledge for decades. Much of the work on concepts in nursing historically was focused on either how to make them clearer or the task of analyzing or synthesizing concepts as a way of developing the knowledge base. Catherine Norris (1982) was one of the first persons to focus on concepts in the context of the nursing knowledge base with her text *Concept Clarification in Nursing*. The work of Walker and Avant (1988, 1995, 2011) is included in many courses oriented toward a discussion of theory in nursing. Along with Norris, Walker and Avant presented nurses with ideas about concept analysis and ushered in a particular focus on analysis that continues decades later. Chinn and Kramer (1991, 2011) also addressed concepts in their writings, particularly with regard to concept development, and it is worth noting that later editions of the popular theory text authored by Meleis (1997, 2012) included a discussion of concepts and the role of concepts in the knowledge base of nursing.

The most common discussions of concepts in nursing since the 1980s, and continuing to the present, have involved the idea of concepts as "building blocks of theory" and, related to that, an emphasis on analysis of concepts (King, 1988). With regard to analysis, a myriad of publications have presented the results of analyses of concepts using diverse approaches and with varying levels of rigor. Although an extensive array of concepts has been addressed in this manner, and multiple analyses have been performed for many concepts, little effort has been expended to tie the analyses to substantive epistemic, scientific, or clinical problems in the discipline or to relate this content to teaching and learning. As a result, the literature abounds with articles on concepts and attempts to clarify concepts with minimal connection to how such approaches solve actual problems or enhance the knowledge base of the discipline (Rodgers, 1989, 2000). Because of the renewed emphasis on concepts in the context of the conceptual approach in nursing education, addressing the discussion of concepts in a more substantive manner is imperative.

WHAT IS A CONCEPT?

A thorough discussion of concepts can go in numerous directions, because concepts have many roles in human existence. As noted previously, concepts are major components of knowledge, theoretical constructions, and organizational tools for thinking. They also can be creative elements, ideas or mental images, essential components of communication, and parts of larger theories. All of these foci point not only to the critical nature of concepts in human cognition and learning but also to the many different roles and uses of concepts that need to be considered to develop a clear understanding of what a concept is.

In general, and from a knowledge standpoint, a concept is "an abstraction that is expressed in some form" (Rodgers, 1989, p. 332), which may seem like a rather simple statement to reflect the essential nature of concepts and the many roles that they play in human existence. Yet this idea of being abstract and being linked to some form of expression is at the core of the definition of "concept." In general, concepts are formed as people encounter different situations and begin to see similarities in those encounters. As a result, the mind forms images that include those common characteristics and the person also learns what word goes along with those images.

MISCONCEPTIONS AND CLARIFICATIONS

Misconception: A concept is something that can be seen or directly measured.

Clarification: Although some concepts can be represented by a physical object, many concepts do not have a corresponding physical object and are represented by ideas, abstractions, mental images, or other modalities.

A child learning what is meant by the word "dog" is a simple example of this process. The child might live with a retriever, visit a family that has a terrier, and have a neighbor with a poodle. The child will hear the word "dog" used to refer to those animals. In a short amount of time the child recognizes that these creatures have some things in common and that the word "dog" does not refer to any specific animal but is applicable to an array of animals that have certain characteristics in common. Hearing the word "dog" stimulates a mental image or idea—that is, the concept of *Dog* that has been formed from a composite of those common characteristics. "Goofy" would be an example of a proper name for a specific dog; "dog" is the term used to express an idea of general characteristics common to all dogs. In conversation, someone might say, "I have a dog," and the person to whom he or she is speaking will immediately know something about the animal to which the original speaker is referring even if that animal is not present during the conversation. The concept that is stimulated on hearing the word "dog" does not specify the type of dog, age, size, or activity level; rather, each individual may have a distinct concept of *Dog* based on experience, familiarity, exposure, and even preference. In spite of individual variation in interpretation, however, everyone involved will be able to converse about these creatures because each has a functional concept of *Dog*. This example shows how the grasping of a concept, based on recognition of common characteristics, makes it possible to refer to something that is not present, to understand such references, and to understand each other and carry on meaningful communication (Rodgers, 2000). It is also evident, based on this example, how learning, or developing a grasp of particular concepts, makes it possible to carry that concept to different situations and conversations and perhaps to new encounters with different dogs. Without concepts, it is not possible to navigate the world, to communicate about it, or to make good decisions about actions.

Concepts also are developed in a person in other ways because not all concepts have physical examples such as *Dog* to facilitate their learning. Concepts such as *Dignity*, *Personhood*, *Grief*,

Health, *Vulnerability*, and *Resilience* are very important in nursing yet do not have corresponding objects that can be pointed to as examples of these concepts. Such concepts are developed through exposure to ideas, human creativity, storytelling, and other modalities. They also are developed through contact with examples and by having the opportunity to experience situations in which the concept exists, even if those situations are not specifically related to the concept on a one-to-one basis, as is the case with physical objects. Nondiscursive forms of presentation are important in learning such concepts, for example, experiential learning or exposure to the arts which provide opportunities to explore concepts in ways that extend beyond verbal discussion.

Concepts are acquired in different ways, but, as the previous example indicates, socialization can be an important part of the process. If the child is only exposed to small dogs, the concept will be constructed on the basis of that exposure and familiarity. The child who later encounters a Great Dane or Mastiff might find that his or her initial concept of *Dog* is challenged and will have to reevaluate, or learn in a new way, that these situations are also appropriate for application of the concept of *Dog*. This has important implications for a conceptual approach to teaching, bringing attention to the way in which the students are exposed to examples of various concepts and the array of variations in application. The concept of *Dignity*, for example, could be discussed with reference to an accomplished and successful individual with impeccable grace and manner, someone who might be referred to as very dignified. *Dignity*, however, also pertains to someone such as an older adult who is hospitalized and unable to participate in self-care or allowed to make decisions. Such treatment might be considered to not respect the dignity of that person. A full grasp of *Dignity* is facilitated by addressing the range of possible applications and variations in use of the concept.

A similar socialization process is at work with other types of concepts, and the profound influence of context is evident in numerous examples in nursing. Many of the concepts that are crucial to the work of nurses do have tangible examples to facilitate learning; an example is the concept of *Sphygmomanometer*. When the student has a grasp of that concept, he or she will understand the idea of the sphygmomanometer whether it is an older mercury tube model, an aneroid model, or an electronic variation. Note that the concept of something is not the object itself. Distinctions exist between (1) the *concept* of *Sphygmomanometer*—that is, the mental or cognitive "idea" about such a tool (an implement of various types that is used to measure blood pressure because it can detect the pressure of the blood against the arterial wall), (2) the *object* sphygmomanometer (that sphygmomanometer over there or one that is physically present), and (3) the *term*, "sphygmomanometer" (i.e., the word that is used to express the concept). The student will have to learn how to operate the specific model, but upon knowing that it is a sphygmomanometer, he or she will immediately know its use in a patient care situation. Although nursing faculty probably think about concepts most often in terms of more abstract ideas, this example shows how conceptual learning actually underlies all learning. If the student learns only about a particular sphygmomanometer, the student will have difficulty when the equipment changes. If the student grasps the concept of *Sphygmomanometer*, the student moves forward with that foundation of learning even when the tool is different. Even when the faculty do not focus on the concept specifically, that type of learning is taking place. Concept-based learning occurs naturally, and sometimes out of view, when the learning environment enables that to occur.

Concepts such as *Dignity*, *Grief*, *Autonomy*, *Quality of Life*, *Safety*, *Patient-centered*, and an abundance of others also are crucial to professional nursing practice, yet no objects exist that can be pointed to as examples of these concepts. In such instances the abstract nature of concepts should be obvious. These examples also make it easy to see how socialization, education, and personal experience and values can influence the particular concept that any nurse holds. Cultural differences in the expression of and norms surrounding many of these concepts are documented extensively. *Grief* is a particularly good example of how norms vary in the formation of a concept (Cowles & Rodgers, 2000), and the value and expressions of autonomy vary with age, gender, and other demographic factors. Many other concepts used in nursing and health care are specific to professionals. *Health Literacy*, for example, is not a concept that the recipients of care generally work with or possess; it is a concept used by the care providers to address an aspect of understanding and involvement in care. An interesting challenge that nurses face is when the recipients of care have different concepts although may be using the same terminology. A patient's concept of autonomy may be very different from that of the nurse, in spite of the fact that both are using the same words. Everyone who has ever been involved in a conversation and thought they were being perfectly clear can appreciate the fact that words and concepts are not always the same across different individuals. Individual meanings may differ as well, and it is important to note that concepts have both definitions (the set of attributes that constitute the concept) and meaning (the values, experience, and personal interpretation an individual has that accompanies the definition). All of these aspects have implications for both teaching and assessment of learning that are discussed throughout this book.

MISCONCEPTIONS AND CLARIFICATIONS

Misconception: Defining a concept is the same as defining how a word is used or stating the meaning of the word.

Clarification: The definition of the concept is the attributes that are clustered together to form the concept. Then a word or term is used to communicate the concept. The concept is the idea or the thinking that is expressed using the word. Meaning is the individual, personal interpretation that a person places on the concept. It is an important part of learning, but it is not the same as definition.

WHY ARE CONCEPTS IMPORTANT?

This discussion about concept acquisition, behavior, and language reveals why concepts are important and are an appropriate focal point in education. Concepts are the objects of thought, and they are organizational elements for thinking. Because of common understandings of language, it is possible to communicate our ideas and concepts with others. It is important to recognize, however, that although different people might use the same word to describe a situation, it does not mean that they possess the same concept. In working with learners, it is important to determine appropriate means of assessment beyond the proper use of a word. It is necessary to evaluate the thinking that underlies that term, in other words, the underlying concept. Nonetheless, without a connection between concepts and some form of expression, most commonly a formal language, communication is not possible. Similarly, without some connection between concepts and action, behavior and actions become random, isolated, and based on a case or situation, without the ability to apply knowledge across different situations. The critical point to remember is that the formation of concepts is essential to learning and to learned action; part of the purpose of learning is to promote in the learner the development of concepts that are relevant, effective, and of practical use.

The previous discussion likely challenges prevailing thinking in nursing about concepts being primarily the "building blocks of theory." This statement is found widely throughout nursing theory texts, and it is generally true when it comes to theory. Unfortunately, this emphasis leaves a lot of people thinking of concepts only in terms of theory, thus ignoring the critical role they play in learning overall. It makes sense that, if concepts are how people think, then they would have a role in theory development. In the conceptual approach to teaching and learning, however, the emphasis is placed on concepts at the level of individual learning rather than in regard to theory in general. This conceptual learning might then be tied to broader theories; for example, an understanding of the concept of *Self-Care* might be tied to broader theories about *Self-Care, Self-management,* or even *Chronic illness.* It should be clear, then, how the conceptual approach not only enhances learning and connects knowledge to action, but creates a logical linkage to a broader theory base to inform nursing practice. Concepts are not merely words but collections of characteristics abstracted from reality, and they typically contain the values, experiences, and socialization of the person who possesses the concepts, which makes them not only essential components of knowledge but powerful tools for effective action.

A Deeper Look at Concepts

The previous discussion of concepts was focused on a general overview of what concepts are and how they are linked to learning, language and action. Some additional discussion of concepts can be helpful in understanding some otherwise subtle differences in how concepts are viewed. The educator using the conceptual approach will benefit from a solid understanding of the nature of concepts and the various aspects of concepts and influences on their development to create appropriate learning experiences and assessments. Problems with implementation of the conceptual approach often can be traced to misunderstanding about what concepts are and how they function. Although this philosophical background may be less interesting than moving forward with application, it is important in order to implement this approach to teaching well and with the desired outcomes for students. Just as students are expected to understand basic physiology before managing the variations that come from disease, this deeper understanding of concepts will facilitate better implementation of the conceptual approach.

A discussion of the nature of concepts can be found throughout a large volume of literature in numerous disciplines. Philosophers have discussed concepts with regard to the study of knowledge (epistemology) and the role that concepts play in the formation of knowledge. In addition to this epistemic focus, philosophers also have explored modes of communication and language (linguistic philosophy), which includes discussion of concepts, and analytic philosophy has been focused on concepts with regard to their relationships to both sentence structure and correspondence with reality. Sociologists have discussed concepts as indicators of societies and group behavior, in addition to the role of concepts and conceptual problems in their own discipline (Lizardo, 2013; Sundbo, 2013), and anthropologists have undertaken similar work in areas related to culture and acculturation. Cognitive psychologists also rely on an understanding of concepts in explanations of learning and knowledge acquisition (Mahon & Caramazza, 2009).

The term "concept" also appears in the literature of other fields with slightly different uses. In the literature of business, references to "concepts" for marketing or product innovation are distinct from the epistemic or knowledge-oriented "concepts" of interest in curriculum development. Yet even this use points to the cognitive or mental aspect of concept formation—that is, creating in the minds of consumers a particular idea about a product and the need for the latest innovation. New products also can lead to new behaviors, as anyone who has witnessed the pre- and post-personal computer era has experienced (Rodgers, 2000). All of these examples indicate that concepts, regardless of focus, constitute an important component of knowledge, learning, socialization, and human existence.

AMBIGUITY ABOUT CONCEPTS

In spite of extensive writing in numerous disciplines, a long history of emphasis on concepts in education, and the recent resurgence of interest in concepts as a focus of teaching, some vagueness exists concerning a number of details about concepts. In spite of a common general understanding of what concepts are, there is some debate specifically about how they are formed in the mind, how shared meanings can develop, how concepts can be taught, what the role of socialization is in the development of individual concepts and collections of concepts, and how the possession or grasp of a particular concept affects behavior and action. In the case of nursing and education, the need to understand how concepts can be taught and how deeper understanding can be developed in students is particularly pressing so the students can acquire the knowledge necessary to perform at a high level. The challenge is much greater than immediate learning, however, because the competent nurse must continue to learn and be willing to change his or her knowledge and behaviors based on changes in knowledge and concepts, and then he or she must demonstrate the application of changes in knowledge through changes in practice. Nurses whose knowledge and actions are limited by context and who are static or unresponsive to new discoveries are not performing in a manner that is consistent with the standards of professional nursing practice. This foundation for continual development needs to be a part of the implementation of the conceptual approach to teaching and learning.

An additional concern involves determining the concepts that are essential to nursing knowledge and how those concepts delineate nursing as a discipline. If nursing education is going to be based on a conceptual approach, a rich understanding regarding concepts in general is needed, along with agreement on a core of concepts that are essential to characterize nursing as a discipline and to provide a substantive basis for reasoned nursing action. The concepts that are selected as the focus for nursing education send a message to students about the core areas of emphasis in the discipline. How those concepts are organized, the language used to communicate them, and the values that are expressed when a concept is shared with students have a considerable impact not only on the learning that takes place but also on the socialization of students to the profession of nursing.

In nursing, concepts often are discussed with an emphasis on their role in theory development, as noted previously. This idea, although widespread in the literature of nursing, will create problems when developing a concept-based curriculum because it gives the impression that theory is needed to link the concepts together to have a sensible and useful knowledge base. Although the value of theory cannot be disputed, concepts themselves are powerful theoretical packages on their own. They can be combined into constructs or into theories, but even when that step is not taken, they are very powerful elements of knowledge all on their own. Even a simple concept such as *Dog* provides a powerful tool to understand these common creatures and their array of sizes and personalities. Consistent with the definition provided earlier that concepts are clusters of characteristics of a phenomenon or experience (Rodgers, 2000), concepts develop through experience—either physical, simulated, or created in the mind—through a process of abstraction from experience. The emphasis on thinking or cognition is common throughout discussions of concepts and is found in the literature of nursing as well, in which authors describe concepts as "mental pictures" or "mental images" (Watson, 1979), words or labels (Diers, 1979; Meleis, 1991), or a combination of these (Hardy, 1974). Each approach has strong implications for concept-based curricula and the teaching and learning of concepts in the discipline. Yet none of these approaches alone is sufficient to explain the role of concepts in the discipline or in human cognition and to provide a foundation for curriculum development and the learning of concepts as part of nursing education. Additional exploration of discussions of concepts in the discipline of philosophy can provide more insight into how concepts function as a component of a discipline's knowledge base.

PHILOSOPHICAL VIEWS OF CONCEPTS

In the literature of philosophy, concepts generally are viewed in one of two distinct ways, each of which has significant implications for the conceptual approach in nursing. The two major traditions in the discussion of concepts have become known as the "entity view" and the "dispositional view." Each of these views has a unique philosophical perspective with regard to what concepts are, how they are formed, and what purpose they serve relative to the external world. It is therefore reasonable that each viewpoint would lead to different approaches in the teaching and learning of nursing concepts. Implications for curriculum development and teaching will be discussed after these different philosophical perspectives are explored.

Table 2.1 ■ **A Comparison of Entity and Dispositional Views of Concepts**

In entity views, the concept	In dispositional views, the concept
• Is composed of necessary and sufficient conditions that are absolute (Essentialism) • Has clear boundaries • Adheres to strict rules of use • Corresponds with an actual object or thing • Is associated with a distinct idea or mental image that enables labeling and categorization • Corresponds to real objects that share the same features • Corresponds to a particular word	• Is composed of attributes that may be fluid or fuzzy (Probabilism) • May show some variation across contexts • Examples have some features in common but may not be identical • Is associated with a mental image that may enables certain competencies related to the concept • Exemplars serve as protoypes rather than absolutes • May be expressed using different words

Entity Views of Concepts

In simple terms, positions consistent with an entity view consider concepts to be *things* (entities), and, consistent with most philosophers who espouse such a review, these things are *ideas* in the mind. Variations of entity views were prevalent in early discussions of concepts that can be found in the literature. Typical of those discussions was attention to concepts as mental objects or images that captured broadly applicable or universal characteristics that are found in the physical world. For example, Aristotle (1947, 1984) discussed concepts as universal essences and gave examples such as *Justice* and *Beauty*; no specific objects can be pointed to about which someone can say, "*that* is 'justice'" or "*there* is 'beauty.'" In other words, justice or beauty cannot be evaluated or determined based on the concept corresponding to a physical object. According to this view, however, some external reference exists against which the concept can be judged—that is, the examples of justice or beauty that exist in the real world. Concepts exist in the mind as objects of thinking according to an entity view, but these concepts relate to examples that can be found in physical reality.

Other prominent philosophers who referred to concepts as ideas include Descartes (1644/1960), Locke (1690/1975), and Kant (1781/1965). Although their discussions of concepts in the mind were considerably different, they all focused on concepts as some component of thought. One implication of this philosophical approach with an emphasis on concepts as being in the mind is that concepts can only be evaluated through some means to get inside the mind to examine these objects of thought. Because that is not possible, these philosophical approaches provide no insight into how to evaluate conceptual learning. In fairness to these philosophers, their focus was on the development of knowledge and the acquisition or ascertainment of truth and not on concept development. Thus a focus of their work and writing was on addressing questions related to the connection between physical reality, the workings of the mind, and the development of knowledge.

In spite of the challenge posed by the apparent need to "get inside the mind" to evaluate the concepts held by a person, entity views did provide a basic answer to the critical question about what a concept is. Throughout entity approaches, concepts are addressed as being composed of attributes that are clustered together to capture characteristics that are common in similar objects or occurrences. This notion of concept persists to the present day and is consistent across most discussions of concepts. What varies is not the answer to what a concept *is* but the many other aspects of concepts, including learning, development, the nature of concepts in the context of a discipline of nursing, and the communication or sharing of concepts.

In the mid-twentieth century, the focus of discussions of concepts in philosophy shifted from the contents within the mind to an emphasis on language. Philosophers in this era showed a particular interest in how language functioned, particularly in their desire to construct an ideal language that would correspond with reality. Philosophers of this tradition, including Frege (1952a, 1952b) and Wittgenstein (in his earlier writings, 1921/1981), viewed concepts essentially as words that should behave in a very specific way relative to the rules of language (see Frege's writings for a discussion of concepts as predicates). For some philosophers of this genre, the emphasis on language and on correspondence was so critical that a word was not considered to be meaningful unless it did correspond to some object.

The implications of this approach are easy to see with regard to concepts that relate to physical objects. For example, nurses learn about thermometers as part of their education, and an actual physical object exists that can be held in the nurse's hand and is referred to using the term "thermometer." In this case, the word "thermometer" is the proper name of such an object. There also is the concept of *Thermometer* that is not any specific thermometer but is an idea the nurse possesses about any number of similar physical objects. They do not all have to look the same or, if electronic or digital, have the same functions and features; the name "thermometer" also can be applied to digital thermometers, glass thermometers, and aural thermometers, for example. However, if the nurse grasps the concept of *Thermometer*, in other words, recognizes the cluster of characteristics, abstracted from the physical objects and representative of all items that can be referred to as "thermometer," the nurse can understand the function and basic operation of any such device. Because such physical objects do exist, the teacher might evaluate the individual's concept by determining whether the learner can identify related objects successfully (i.e., thermometers), communicate about them, and differentiate thermometers from other devices. Correspondence works, to a certain extent, with an array of concepts for which there are representative physical objects.

Although the example concerning the concept of *Thermometer* is straightforward, concepts that are important in nursing (and in life in general) often pertain to nonphysical occurrences, as is the case with the concepts of *Professional* or *Dignity* (or *Justice* and *Beauty*, *Grief*, and many others). These concepts share the same origin in being formed on the basis of a cluster of characteristics or attributes. Although there is not a physical object that can be pointed to as "professional," there are experiences with examples of these concepts that can be provided through the educational process and by way of role modeling and observation. The nurse, or nursing student, can develop a grasp of the concept of *Professional* through these encounters and thus have a broader understanding rather than knowledge that is based on specific cases or situations. It does not serve the student well if he or she can only point to a particular person as being *Professional* or not, or someone who acts in a *Professional* manner. Instead, students need to understand what it is to be *Professional* and then be able to apply that across a variety of circumstances. This surely seems like a very abstract idea, but it is the difference between understanding how to label something and treating words as names or in grasping the abstract learning that guides that use of words.

This critical function of concepts has an important role in nursing education. For some philosophers, such as Frege and the early writings of Wittgenstein, concepts that lacked corresponding objects were considered to be without meaning. Concepts such as *Justice*, *Dignity*, *Autonomy*, and many more that are critical not only to nursing but in human existence could not meet this requirement for correspondence. In nursing, there is a tendency to struggle with how to promote learning of these concepts. It is easier, sometimes, to work with things that can be seen, touched, or heard. But much of what is important in nursing cannot be seen or touched, and that content needs to be a part of student learning as well. In fact, the conceptual approach helps to put that type of information on the same footing as more tangible aspects of nursing knowledge. All that is needed is for the teacher to recognize that much of learning actually is conceptual in nature, even for those things that have related physical objects.

Research supports some of the challenges with entity views of concepts. Particularly important with regard to concept-based teaching and learning is research in psychology, which raises significant questions about whether the way human beings form concepts is consistent with an entity view (Armstrong, Gleitman, & Gleitman, 1983; Fehr, 1988; McCloskey & Glucksberg, 1978; Medin, 1989; Medin & Schaffer, 1978; Rodgers, 2000; Smith & Medin, 1981). As quickly becomes evident in implementing the conceptual approach, determining the critical characteristics of a concept can be very challenging. Assessment of learning is another area of challenge. The Entity view requires a very strict interpretation of the definition of the concept, in other words, the attributes that constitute the definition of the concept. There is no mechanism for judging or weighting that allows one exemplar to be considered a better example than another. The concept of *Health* provides a good example of the variation that exists and many concepts in nursing are subject to strong individual differences and perceptions. Numerous examples of the concept of *Health* could be presented and, depending on the person being asked, some instances would appear to be better examples than others or would appear to be examples that serve as better prototypes. Nurses are quite familiar with how "health" can be defined very differently by different people based on experience, goals, values, history, and context. Yet examples are sure to exist that are stronger or clearer for many concepts and that provide better examples for teaching purposes, and the faculty would expect a student to recognize such examples. According to an entity view, individual perceptions are not relevant in the definition of a concept and in the identification of instances of a particular concept. Perhaps this characteristic points to one of the most troublesome aspects of an entity view, in that it is not consistent with how people learn and function as members of interactive societies. The challenges with this view can alert the teacher to the pitfall of being too rigid in the definition of a concept. Students need to be able to work with the appropriate degree of variation to facilitate flexibility in their learning and the ability to use the concept effectively in different situations.

Dispositional Views of Concepts

Presenting a stark contrast to entity approaches to concepts are what are called dispositional theories of concepts. In entity views, a concept is considered to be objects or specific things that could be examined and evaluated on their own. In a dispositional view, a concept is regarded as a behavior or, more specifically, a capability for a particular behavior. From the perspective of the entity view, evaluation of whether or not someone has a grasp of the concept is focused on exploring that actual concept—the definition, rules, and conditions that make up the concept. Applying this to the concept of *Dog*, the entity view requires that the individual be able to list the attributes appropriately so as to have the specific "right" concept of *Dog*. In a dispositional view, the individual would be expected to determine what is or is not a dog, to use the word "dog" appropriately, and to act in an appropriate way when an example of *Dog* is present. Even for concepts related to physical objects, such as *Dog*, the advantages to the dispositional view are clear for the conceptual approach to teaching. It is not enough to just be able to list the attributes, especially because there is usually some fuzziness about those in defining the concept. The person who has a good grasp of the concept is able to act on that knowledge in a way that is appropriate to show an accurate or functional understanding. An application to nursing can be seen using the concept of *Bacteria*, just to give one example.

In a dispositional view, concepts are abstractions, not things themselves. The concept of *Bacteria* is not actual bacteria; the concept is a cognitive development that arises based on an understanding of bacteria on an abstract level—in other words, some characteristics that bacteria have in common. The individual who grasps the idea or concept of *Bacteria* will learn that the word "bacteria" is used to express that concept and, as such, can talk about these things using the word properly. According to dispositional views, a solid grasp of a concept enables a person to do more than communicate; the person who understands the concept also is able to perform in certain ways. The nurse who possesses a strong grasp of the concept of *Bacteria* will be able to understand the differences between bacteria and viruses and the role of antibiotics in management, along with the role of other nursing interventions such as handwashing and isolation techniques. Similarly, a nurse who has a strong grasp of the concept of *Health* will be able to identify things that are examples of health and act in suitable ways (for example, in the promotion of health, assuming that health promotion is a desirable goal). These examples provide a clear picture of some of the strengths of dispositional views, not just in a discipline such as nursing but in everyday life. Health is not a single object; rather, it is something that can be present in varying degrees and in widely different ways in different people and contexts. Health is something that tends to exist more or less. Although it may be possible to identify, or at least construct, a single outstanding example of "health," being able to say about a particular instance "this is health" and "this is not health" is not realistic and is not likely to be functional in practical application. There is no single thing that goes by the name "health" that could match a concept of *Health* as needed in an entity view. Dispositional theories include attention to the behaviors that are possible when someone has a grasp of a concept rather than just the ability to identify what is and is not a corresponding object. Concepts have had a major role in human understanding of learning, science, and knowledge development. A deeper understanding of the role of concepts, as well as insight into the history of changing views, can review the works of some of the leading philosophers in this area, including Hallett (1967), Hartnack (1965), Ryle (1949, 1971a-d), and Wittgenstein (1953/1968, 1968).

HOW CLEAR CAN OUR CONCEPTS BE?

Another important aspect of concepts that stems from philosophical differences can be very confusing for the faculty using the conceptual approach. This aspect concerns how rigid and clear in definition a concept is required to be. When concepts are confused with words or specific objects, the tendency will be to think of the concept as having a very clear and rigid definition. Assessment of learning, then, might be focused on whether the student has things "right" in terms of being able to define or explain the concept. Although all views of concepts focus on the attributes that compose the concept, the extent to which these are specific, clear, or unchanging does vary. Certainly some definitions of concepts are more acceptable or more accurate than others, and some are way off base so as to be determined that the student does not have a good grasp of the concept. But it is important for the faculty member to recognize that many concepts, if not most, will have a little bit of fuzziness that needs to be accommodated and understood when talking about concepts. Concepts represent a continuum, with varying degrees of abstractness that affect how they are learned and applied.

Philosophers refer to this as the *contrast of essentialism and probabilism.* Looking again at the example of the concept of *Dog,* as with all concepts, this concept is composed of the characteristics that are present in order to think appropriately about something using the concept and its associated label, "dog." There are certain things that need to be present to consider something to be an example of "dog." There are other things that may also be present that are not required for the example to fit the concept of *Dog*. Although this may seem particularly simplistic (after all, everyone knows what a dog is, it seems), it also is easy to see how determining boundaries can be more difficult than might be imagined. Consider, for example, a hyena, jackal, coyote, or other similar animal that looks a lot like what generally is considered to be a "dog," what seems to fit our concept of *Dog* quite easily, but is usually not referred to using the concept and associated term "dog." So what are these creatures? At what point does *Dog* no longer apply and something else does as the relevant concept?

An essentialist position argues that those boundaries are actually very rigid and clear. Something either is appropriately referenced using the concept of *Dog,* or the relevant attributes are not there, and it is not an example of *Dog*. Essentialism, with regard to concepts, means that the attributes are both necessary and sufficient to define the concept. If any aspect is missing, the situation is not an example of that concept. Easy enough. Except when it is not, as the case of coyote, for example, makes clear. A probabilistic view focuses on a core of attributes that are *generally* required, but there is a bit of fuzziness that allows for some judgment as well as acknowledge that concepts evolve over time as new evidence emerges (Figure 2-2). For example, a *germ,* in the context of human health, in very general terms is an organism capable of causing disease. But what has been learned about germs, how they cause disease, how they get transmitted, etc., has changed significantly since the early knowledge about germs and germ theory. It is important that students be encouraged to examine their thinking and recognize the potential for change and for expansion to set the foundation for lifelong learning. A very rigid approach to concepts and the learning of concepts is more likely to promote a system of rote learning that is not conducive to lifelong learning.

One place where a more rigid form of definition seems for functional is in the area of taxonomies. The more rigid end of that continuum is anchored by concepts that have been constructed and stipulated by humans and that do have very specific criteria that are either present, or not, to be an example of the concept. Taxonomies are good examples of these constructed concepts. Because the definitions are stipulated, with very precise criteria, a different type of learning may be facilitated and faculty might expect more stringent application of criteria. Many disease categories as well have strict criteria that determine whether the specific diagnosis applies. It is also possible, however, that there is some conflict

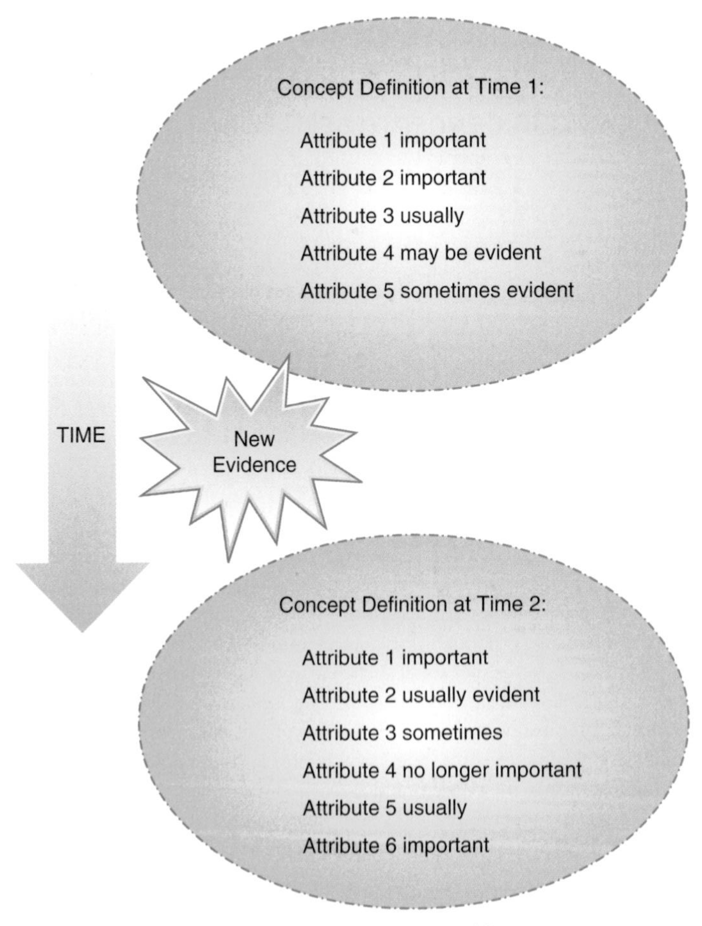

Fig. 2.2 Concepts evolve over time as new evidence emerges.

between the underlying concept and the concept as it appears in a taxonomic listing. A nurse may have a clear concept of *Dementia,* but this may not be exactly the same as a diagnosis of dementia. This just presents another example of how concepts, words, taxonomies all can vary. With conceptual learning, the emphasis on the concept provides the critical foundation on which it is possible to build word use, diagnoses, and other related ideas. A good grasp and understanding of the concept provides an organizing structure to understand taxonomies, diagnoses, and variations of the condition being addressed.

As the example of dementia demonstrates, the clarity and rigidity of the essentialist view may seem desirable, but it may also be an illusion. Even in the case of taxonomies, which involve strictly prescribed definitions, there can be challenges in the attempt to create categories that are mutually exclusive and without overlap. In some fields this task is easier to achieve, such as in the classification of biologic organisms (e.g., flowers or insects). In situations involving humans, however, criteria often are presented in the form of a list in which only some of the items on the list must be present for the label to be applicable, thus indicating that there is no single core of characteristics that is captured by the concept. Diagnostic categories change on the basis of new knowledge and changes in social norms, and thus these taxonomies must be reconstructed periodically. Autism is a good example of a situation in which considerable change has occurred over time, resulting in the evolution of the concept to become *Autism Spectrum Disorder.* Taxonomies often function according the idea that it is possible to identify the attributes or characteristics of the concept and that these attributes or characteristics comprise a set of "necessary and sufficient conditions," including conditions that must be present (are necessary) and that together are enough (are sufficient) to warrant the taxonomic label. In this example, even with constructed taxonomies that are highly structured, a little bit of fuzziness is necessary. This realization points out the importance of judgment and good decision making in the application of the concept. Perhaps a concept related to a diagnosis requires three things to be present and one or more of another list. Anyone who has worked with human beings knows that there are always some situational variations, gaps in the history that people provide about a condition, or some things that are more or less present with lots of gray areas. Conceptual learning brings not only the concepts that underlie learning to the forefront but the thinking and decision-making that is critical to good nursing practice as well. The conceptual approach is not just about the concepts but about using the concepts, applying them, making decisions about them, and then acting on the basis of a solid foundational system organized around a cohesive system of concepts.

What Does This Mean for Concept-Based Teaching?

Effective teaching using the conceptual approach requires an understanding of the different perspectives that exist about concepts. The assumptions that are made about the nature of concepts and their role in the discipline affect the teaching strategies that are used in a concept-based approach to nursing education. The previous discussion reveals some of the array of approaches that exist in philosophy and how those approaches may affect or be manifested in nursing education. This deeper thought regarding the nature of concepts, how they are acquired, what purposes they serve, and how they manifest and are expressed is essential to avoid significant pitfalls that can hinder the learning process and make the conceptual approach less fulfilling, and more frustrating, for teacher and students. Some of the areas in which confusion is particularly likely to be troublesome are described in the following section.

CLARITY REGARDING TERMINOLOGY

At the most basic level, clarity about terminology is important. Faculty who teach any curriculum need to be clear in how they use words to describe certain phenomena. This clarity is particularly critical when talking about areas that are replete with ambiguity and confusion, as is the case with theoretical ideas such as concepts. The definition given previously, that concepts are clusters of attributes that are abstracted from phenomena and given an associated term for expression, is simple, complete, and broadly applicable to concepts of all types (Rodgers, 2000). It is also, however, not likely to be something most faculty have considered. Again, the emphasis here is on concepts and conceptual thinking as the foundation of a conceptual approach to teaching and learning.

Concepts are thoughts or ideas that are expressed using words; they are not the words themselves. Concepts also are not objects and need to be differentiated from specific objects and also from measurement devices such as research or physical instruments. Instruments, tools, and physical implements used in nursing are mechanisms to measure abstract concepts. A thermometer is a tool to measure an aspect of *Thermoregulation,* with *Thermoregulation* being the concept of interest. In teaching, it is important to be distinct about the abstract idea (concept) and the physical manifestation of that concept. *Thermometer* also can be a concept—that is, the concept of *Thermometer,* or the general idea of something that is used to measure temperature—if discussion is about thermometers in general. So, there is the idea, the object, and this is followed by desired action, the ability to use a thermometer properly to measure (and interpret) temperature. Someone who grasps the concept of *Thermometer* will be able to use any of a variety of types of thermometers appropriately. This may seem very simplistic, but apply this same process to the concept of *Dyspnea.* Understanding the concept enables the individual who grasps the concept to identify, interpret, and take action based on a solid understanding of dyspnea wherever that occurs across the lifespan and health spectrum. Awareness of the distinction between concept, word, and object is critical to effective concept-based teaching.

CONCEPTS AND CONSTRUCTS

Concepts also can be clustered to form constructs. When teaching and developing curricula, it is important to recognize the base elements—that is, the simplest concepts—along with what are more properly regarded as constructs. Concept-based teaching may be focused on both. For example, *Thermoregulation* includes the concepts of *Regulation,* as well as concepts related to *Temperature, Heat, Cold,* and *Measurement.* In most cases, constructs can be addressed in teaching in the same manner as concepts. However, it may be helpful to address the basic elements of such constructs to assist students in learning.

CONCEPTS AND CONTEXT

Concepts also are combined, sometimes, into theory. A common misconception in nursing is based on the often-repeated statement that "concepts are the building blocks of theory" (Rodgers & Knafl, 2000). Although this statement is true, theories are constructed through the identification of relationships among concepts, and this ubiquitous statement gives the impression that concepts are not of value unless they are in the context of theory. The theoretical literature in nursing is focused on the weaving together of concepts to make theory. What is lost in this process is the recognition that concepts themselves have value and are, to some extent, theoretical products. As is evident in the discussion of philosophy earlier in this chapter, concepts are very powerful theoretical elements that carry with them the influences of society, history, culture, disciplines, and existing knowledge. In other words, concepts are contextually bound. Attempts to view them as universal or as the same regardless of context will undermine a primary value of nursing with regard to the uniqueness of each individual. There is such a thing as the concept of *Health.* What will be considered to be the attributes of the concept of *Health,* and thus suitable examples of the concept, will vary widely across contexts. Using the previous example of the concept of *Dyspnea,* dyspnea has certain characteristics (attributes) that make it dyspnea regardless of setting. The context, however, will introduce other variations, as well as indicate what actions are warranted to fully assess and then intervene appropriately.

THE NEED FOR A CONSISTENT PHILOSOPHICAL APPROACH

Consistency in the philosophical approach to concepts that underlie a concept-based curriculum can be very helpful to students as they proceed with their conceptual learning. It is tempting at times to see some concepts as static, with clear boundaries, and with obvious and clear examples of appropriate use. It certainly makes teaching and assessment of learning easier if that is the case. Yet it is obvious in some of the previous examples that this approach does not fit the majority of concepts. Although some concepts have a well-developed and fairly consistent core (the concept of *Dementia,* for example which, if looked at in the context of diagnosis, has certain attributes that are relatively static and required for a diagnosis to be justified), even those have some element of "fuzziness" and potential for change over time. If the faculty consider some concepts to be very rigid with clear and well-defined boundaries and others as fuzzy, that can be confusing to students because it encourages more memorization for those that are rigid and more creative and interpretation for the others. Recognizing that some fuzziness exists for all concepts enables the faculty to present concepts from the same philosophical perspective and promote a more flexible and open type of learning regardless of the subject matter. This is a critical part of a foundation for continual learning throughout the professional career. Even the most concrete of concepts will have some variation either across humans or over time. The possibility and the likelihood of change over time must be acknowledged for all concepts (see Fig 2-2).

Allowing for some flexibility and a dynamic approach to accept the inevitability of change over time, there are some differences in the degree of clarity that exists for concepts across the spectrum. Concepts do occupy a continuum ranging from concrete to abstract, well developed to amorphous, widely fluctuating over time and context to relatively stable. Morse (1995) discussed this idea of stability and clarity with regard to how "mature" the concept is. However, it has nothing to do with maturity or longevity; it has to do with the strength of evidence supporting some concepts. Some aspects of existence are less subject to fluctuation and change than are others. For example, at any point in time there are clear criteria for what constitutes hypertension. These criteria change as the science changes, yet the criteria that result are always clear. In spite of that, there will always be people who present with variation of this otherwise clear condition. Labile hypertension has been considered a separate class, yet evidence indicates that all hypertension shows some lability. Some disease conditions that seem very obvious end up having different origins—for example, the discovery of *Helicobacter pylori* as a causative agent for peptic ulcers. It was "known" with great certainty what caused such ulcers...until the evidence became overwhelming that the widely accepted certainty was not so certain after all.

So, for persons teaching according to concept-based curricula, it is important to be consistent with the view of concepts that underlies the curriculum and with how each instructor or faculty member presents that view in different learning encounters. A defensible view of concepts must allow for processes of conceptual change. In fact, promoting awareness of processes of conceptual change in students can help strengthen a value for keeping up with current literature and discoveries. A shortcoming of education regardless of the approach can be the imparted belief that there is such a thing as proof or "truth"; in the case of concept-based curricula, ample opportunities exist to reinforce the common nature of conceptual change.

Assessment must be consistent with the philosophical view of concepts and the nature of the particular conceptual learning that is being evaluated. Teaching conceptually but testing specific details or "facts" will send a contradictory message to students regarding the importance of conceptual understanding in nursing. It also is likely to skew assessment results because the mode of teaching will not be consistent with the form of evaluation or measurement. Consequently, a critical issue in effective concept-based teaching is the determination of how understanding can be evaluated appropriately, which can vary with the origin, nature, specificity, clarity, and subjective nature of specific concepts.

CONCEPTS GROUNDED IN NURSING DISCIPLINE

Finally, it is important to recognize that concept-based teaching must be grounded in the specific conceptual base of the discipline of nursing. In selecting the concepts to be included in the curriculum, and in discriminating among closely related concepts, students are being socialized into the discipline and profession of nursing (Toulmin, 1972). The concepts that are chosen as the focus for teaching will shape the professional identity and development of the students as Registered Nurses. The role of concept-based teaching in the development of the student as a professional nurse may seem like it places a strong burden on the curriculum and faculty. It is, however, an outstanding opportunity for shaping the future of the discipline.

Summary

The conceptual approach to teaching in nursing offers a number of advantages as an educational model for student learning. It matches an important part of the natural process of learning, provides a foundation and skills for life-long development, creates receptivity and openness to change consistent with a dynamic knowledge base, and emphasizes the knowledge that underlies practice rather than merely the jobs or roles in which nurses perform. For such an approach to be successful, however, it is essential that the faculty have an understanding of the nature of concepts and how they function in the process of learning and be consistent in their philosophical viewpoint about concepts. Faculty also need to recognize the importance of conceptual change in the discipline and connect that to evidence-based practice. Doing so will provide the students not only with a foundation of concepts essential for nursing practice but an appreciation for adapting to new developments in the discipline as they arise. Concepts lose their value if they are seen as static entities to be memorized and matched up with segments of reality. Grasping and applying concepts, and using the appropriate language to express them, is a dynamic process that empowers the students not only to perform at high levels but also to keep current with new developments as they pursue their careers in nursing.

References

Aristotle. Posterior Analytics (Mure GRG, Trans). In: McKeon R, ed. *Introduction to Aristotle*. New York, NY: Random House; 1947:9–109.

Aristotle. Categories (Ackrill JL, Trans). In: Barnes J, ed. *The Complete Works of Aristotle*. Princeton, NJ: Princeton University; 1984:3–24.

Armstrong SL, Gleitman LR, Gleitman H. What some concepts might not be. *Cognition*. 1983;13:263–308.

Chinn PL, Kramer MK. *Theory and Nursing: A Systematic Approach*. 3rd ed. St. Louis, MO: Mosby; 1991.

Chinn PL. *Kramer MK: Integrated Theory and Knowledge Development in Nursing*. 8th ed. St. Louis, MO: Elsevier; 2011.

Cowles KV, Rodgers BL. The concept of grief: an evolutionary perspective. In: Rodgers BL, Knafl KA, eds. *Concept Development in Nursing: Foundations, Techniques, and Applications*. Philadelphia, PA: Saunders; 2000:103–117.

Descartes R. Meditations on first philosophy. In: Beardsley MC, ed. *The European Philosophers from Descartes to Nietzsche*. New York, NY: Random House; 1960:25–96. Original work published 1644.

Diers D. *Research in Nursing Practice*. Philadelphia, PA: J. B. Lippincott; 1979.

Fehr B. Prototype analysis of the concepts of love and commitment. *J Pers Soc Psychol*. 1988;55:557–579.

Frege G. Grundgesetze der Arithmetic (Geach PT, Trans.). In: Geach P, Black M, eds. *Translations from the Philosophical Writings of Gottlob Frege*. Oxford, United Kingdom: Basil Blackwell; 1952:159–181.

Frege G. On concept and object (Geach PT, Trans). In: Geach P, Black M, eds. *Translations from the Philosophical Writings of Gottlob Frege*. Oxford, United Kingdom: Basil Blackwell; 1952:42–55.

Hallett G. *Wittgenstein's Definition of Meaning as Use*. New York, NY: Fordham University; 1967.

Hardy MK. Theories: Components, development, evaluation. *Nurs Res*. 1974;23:100–107.

Hartnack J. *Wittgenstein and Modern Philosophy.* (M. Cranston, Trans.). New York, NY: New York University; 1965.
Kant I. *Critique of Pure Reason (Smith NK, Trans.).* New York, NY: St. Martin's Press; 1965 (Original work published 1781.).
King IM. Concepts: Essential elements of theories. *Nursing Science Quarterly.* 1988;1:22–25.
Lizardo O. Re-conceptualizing abstract conceptualization in social theory: the case of the "structure" concept. *Journal for the Theory of Social Behaviour.* 2013;43(2):155–180.
Locke J. *An Essay Concerning Human Understanding.* Oxford, United Kingdom: Oxford University; 1975 (Original work published 1690.).
Mahon BZ, Caramazza A. Concepts and categories: a cognitive neuropsychological perspective. *Annual Review of Psychology.* 2009;60:27–51.
McCloskey ME, Glucksberg S. Natural categories: Well defined or fuzzy sets? *Memory & Cognition.* 1978;6:462–472.
Medin DL. Concepts and conceptual structure. *American Psychologist.* 1989;44:1469–1481.
Medin DL, Schaffer MM. Context theory of classification learning. *Psychol Rev.* 1978;85:207–238.
Meleis AI. *Theoretical Nursing.* 2nd ed. Philadelphia, PA: J. B. Lippincott; 1991.
Meleis AI. *Theoretical Nursing.* 3rd ed. Philadelphia, PA: J. B. Lippincott; 1997.
Meleis AI. *Theoretical Nursing.* 5th ed. Philadelphia, PA: Lippincott Williams & Wilkins; 2012.
Morse MM. Exploring the theoretical basis of nursing knowledge using advanced techniques of concept analysis. *Adv Nurs Sci.* 1995;17(3):31–46.
Norris CM. *Concept Clarification in Nursing.* Rockville, MD: Aspen; 1982.
Rodgers BL. Concepts, analysis, and the development of nursing knowledge: the evolutionary cycle. *J Adv Nurs.* 1989;14:330–335.
Rodgers BL. Philosophical foundations of concept development. In: Rodgers BL, Knafl KA, eds. *Concept Development in Nursing: Foundations, Techniques, and Applications.* Philadelphia, PA: W. B. Saunders; 2000:7–37.
Rodgers BL, Knafl KA. Introduction to concept development in nursing. In: Rodgers BL, Knafl KA, eds. *Concept Development in Nursing: Foundations, Techniques, and Applications.* Philadelphia, PA: W. B. Saunders; 2000:1–6.
Ryle G. *The Concept of Mind.* Chicago, IL: University of Chicago; 1949.
Ryle G. Systematically misleading expressions. In: *Collected Papers.* vol. 2. London, United Kingdom: Hutchinson; 1971a:39–62.
Ryle G. The theory of meaning. In: *Collected Papers.* vol. 2. London, United Kingdom: Hutchinson; 1971b:350–372.
Ryle G. Thinking thoughts and having concepts. In: *Collected Papers.* vol. 2. London, United Kingdom: Hutchinson; 1971c:446–450.
Ryle G. Use, usage and meaning. In: *Collected Papers.* vol 2. London, United Kingdom: Hutchinson; 1971d:407–414.
Smith EE, Medin DL. *Categories and Concepts.* Cambridge, MA: Harvard University; 1981.
Sundbo DIC. Local food: The social construction of a concept, Section B, Soil and plant science. *Acta Agriculturae Scandinavica B.* 2013;63(sup1):66–77.
Toulmin S. *Human Understanding.* Princeton, NJ: Princeton University; 1972.
Walker LO, Avant KC. *Strategies for Theory Construction in Nursing.* 2nd ed. Norwalk, CT: Appleton & Lange; 1988.
Walker LO, Avant KC. *Strategies for Theory Construction in Nursing.* 3rd ed. Norwalk, CT: Appleton & Lange; 1995.
Walker LO, Avant KC. *Strategies for Theory Construction in Nursing.* 5th ed. Boston, MA: Prentice-Hall; 2011.
Watson J. *Nursing: The Philosophy and Science Of Caring.* Boston, MA: Little, Brown; 1979.
Wittgenstein L. *Philosophical Investigations.* 3rd ed. (G. E. M. Anscombe, Trans.). New York, NY: Macmillan; 1968. (Original work published 1953.)
Wittgenstein L. *Tractatus Logico-Philosophicus.* (D. F. Pears & B. F. McGuinness, Trans.). London, United Kingdom: Routledge & Kegan Paul; 1981. (Original work published 1921.)

CHAPTER 3

Development of Concepts for Concept-Based Teaching

Beth Rodgers

A general overview of ideas associated with concepts as a foundation for understanding the nature and use of concepts and implementing the conceptual approach to teaching was presented in Chapter 2. As described in that chapter, the specific approach that is taken toward concepts has a clear impact on concept-based teaching. It is important that instructors working with the conceptual approach understand the confusion that exists regarding what a concept is, as well as the many different approaches to concepts. The perspective taken by the faculty, and represented by the curriculum overall, can have a profound effect on student learning and on how concept-based teaching and learning occur.

In addition to having a clear idea about what concepts are in general, faculty need to have a shared idea about concepts so as to not confuse students by offering different interpretations. If one faculty member thinks of concepts in terms of words or names of physical objects, this will confuse students and hinder their ability to deal with more abstract ideas. Students in a program that involves a conceptual approach will benefit also if faculty are similar in their approach to promoting acceptance of change in concepts and an appreciation for how new evidence can influence thinking and the practice that follows. Whereas all faculty do not have to be exactly the same, awareness of differences and at least some shared understanding regarding what concepts are and how they are acquired can enhance student progression through the program.

Faculty also will need to determine not only which concepts are relevant to the curriculum but what should be the focus of each aspect of the curriculum in terms of definitions, use, and language. Once those decisions are made, there will be a shared foundation for moving forward with the construction of appropriate learning activities. At that point, faculty members are confronted with a challenging and multifaceted task. For each chosen concept in the curriculum, a number of aspects need to be considered: How does the faculty define and present the concept to students? In what settings do instances of the concept occur? What effect does context/setting/user have on the concept? What other concepts are similar, related, or easily confused with the concept of interest? How is that concept expressed or shared or discussed with others? What means are appropriate to assess a student's grasp of the concept? Other chapters in this text deal with various aspects of these challenges. In this chapter, the focus is on definitions, relationships among concepts, and language, because these components are critical to the formation of learning and assessment strategies as a foundation for developing and implementing a sound curriculum for concept-based teaching.

Defining the Concepts

Nursing faculty are familiar with the common use of the term "definition." Dictionaries of all shapes and sizes are full of definitions that address the common purpose of using a word in a particular way to promote communication. One popular resource provides a definition of *definition*:

BOX 3.1 ■ Homonyms

A homonym is a word with the same spelling and pronunciation but with different definitions. A homonym does not usually express the same *concept*. Each use of the term must be associated with a different concept and conceptual definition for correct application. Consider all the following applications for the concept of *Bill:*

Money; a dollar bill
The part of a bird's jaw with a horny covering; a beak
An itemized statement of fees or charges
The visor portion of a cap
A common first name
A draft of proposed law presented for legislation

"a statement of the exact meaning of a word, especially in a dictionary.... An exact statement or description of the nature, scope, or meaning of something" (*Oxford Dictionary of English*, 2005, p. 455). In simple terms, a definition of a word may be referred to as the "meaning" of that word, similar to its reference or proper use in a sentence. Knowing the definition of a word enables a person to use that word effectively in a sentence and, if the person on the receiving end understands that definition, that individual can understand what the speaker or writer is trying to convey. When the number of homonyms in the English language is considered, the need for definitions of this type becomes clear (Box 3.1). Homonyms also point out the importance of making a distinction between concepts and the words that are used to express those concepts. The words may be the same, but in many cases, the concepts expressed by the word can be very different.

Definitions typically are written as declarative statements and often as sentence fragments, such as the definition of "grief" presented in the *Oxford Dictionary of English* (2005): "intense sorrow, especially caused by someone's death." It also is defined in this same source as "an instance or cause of intense sorrow" (p. 762). Such definitions, when shared, make communication possible on a general level. But they also present a lot of questions that indicate how that communication may not be as common as desired. With regard to developing a knowledge base or using an idea or phenomenon definitively in research or theory, the problems should be obvious. What counts as "intense sorrow"? According to this dictionary, grief is "especially caused by someone's death." Are there other causes? Can intense sorrow stem from some other type of loss? What are the differences between sorrow and anguish, despair, and hopelessness? Do people act out their grief in different ways, and is it still "grief" if the behaviors differ? Such questions reveal how unclear our terminology really is sometimes and the challenges that terminology can present in nursing situations.

Conceptual definitions require a greater degree of specificity. A conceptual definition is not the same as a common definition nor is it the same as meaning. As pointed out in Chapter 2, a concept is composed of a set of attributes. A conceptual definition therefore is a clear statement of those attributes. A definition can be considered adequate, or more appropriately "conceptually adequate," when it stipulates the components of the concept with sufficient clarity that the concept can be used effectively (Rodgers, 2000). As discussed in Chapter 2, all of the attributes may not be particularly stable or certain. There may be a core that is stable over time but some more nuanced aspects that are open to change over time or may show variation across different contexts. Some concepts will have a more stable and specific core of attributes than others. For example, the concept of *Sepsis* can be defined by stating the attributes that are essential to identify, without a doubt, an instance of actual sepsis. This definition should work across a variety of contexts. Although it is highly likely that new evidence will be gained about sepsis over time, this concept has been in existence for a long time and has been fairly consistent, so it is possible to feel confident in its definition. In this case, change is more likely to be seen in terms of science related to risk factors, protective mechanisms, and other aspects that influence the course and outcome of sepsis. The definition of the concept may change in time but generally can be seen as quite stable. A conceptually adequate definition of the concept of *Sepsis,* then, will provide the attributes that are appropriate to recognizing sepsis and understanding the contextual factors that lead to and follow its occurrence.

It is important to differentiate "definition" from "meaning," however, because these two terms are easily confused when discussing concepts. It will be confusing to students to use these terms loosely, so a bit of attention to the difference is needed here. The typical dictionary definition of the word "definition" typically includes a mention of the "meaning" of a word. Meaning, however, can be a much more complex idea. Meaning is not merely a description of how a word can be used but can refer to the personal, emotional, reflective impact of a situation on a person. The definition of *justice* should not be confused with the "meaning" of justice, or the unique, highly nuanced idea that justice has for a particular individual or that may be shared among a group of individuals. Meaning comes from experience, exposure, and personal interaction with events and the development of that personal impact is an important adjunct to learning. Distinguishing definition and meaning provides another opportunity to enrich conceptual learning in students. For example, a student may encounter an individual who is struggling to accept a new diagnosis of type II diabetes and who is having difficulty learning the tasks and changes that will be necessary for healthy management of the condition. Conversations with that patient along with observations of the individual's interaction with other health care personnel reveal that this is an example of the concept of *Self-Management.* The student may know the definition of the concept of *Self-Management* and is able to recognize it in this situation and apply appropriate knowledge about that concept. The student also can be encouraged by the faculty to think about the "meaning" of self-management for this particular individual (and perhaps for the student as well). The definition of the concept of *Self-Management* does not include how particular values might appear in regard to self-management—does that person want to be involved in self-management? Does the individual value self-management or is the history (or the clinical situation) encouraging a more passive approach to care? The student might be encouraged to think about his or her own values and preferences and what it would be like to be in that situation. Recognizing the difference between definition and meaning provides the opportunity for an additional type of learning that enhances the concept-based learning and addresses some of the other domains of learning (affective, aesthetic, for example) that are essential to higher level practice in nursing.

CONCEPTUAL CHANGE OVER TIME

As noted previously, the idea that concepts can be defined by strict criteria that do not change (referred to as *necessary and sufficient conditions*) at first glance does seem to fit some of the ideas that are critical to nursing knowledge (Walker & Avant, 2011). But there are numerous instances where this is not consistent. Furthermore, even for those instances that do seem to fit at present, the possibility and in fact the likelihood of change in the future needs to be instilled in students as a reminder to keep up to date with the latest knowledge. History is full of examples of situations in which there seemed good reason to believe that certainty had been achieved, only to have that certainty questioned over time. A student in astronomy who had a solid grasp of the concept of *Planet* probably was very comfortable with the classification of Pluto as a planet—until it was no longer classified that way. Ultimately, a newer concept of *Dwarf Planet* evolved, all the time building on a general idea of planet, but with the opportunity for change and refinement over time as new information about Pluto and other astronomical bodies was uncovered. The interplay of ideas lead to a different understanding of the concepts of planet and dwarf planet and, of course, the specific planet Pluto. Health care and nursing experience similar changes over time on an ongoing basis and, in fact, this change is essential to reflect emerging science.

As described before, a more defensible view of concepts allows for this evolution and focuses on the use of concepts rather than on correspondence theory as if concepts were just words or names (Rodgers, 2000). This view also is a good fit with concept-based teaching. A student could be very adept at reciting facts and listing details and principles, but if the student cannot apply that knowledge in real-life situations, the learning is of limited or no value. It is the use of concepts that makes it clear whether the student has a full grasp of the essential knowledge. It is not sufficient in nursing to merely "know" something; rather, it is essential that the nurse be able to apply that knowledge, recognize subtle nuances and variations in application across multiple settings and situations, evaluate the application, and alter that knowledge based on evaluation and as new quality information becomes available. The approach to concepts and concept-based teaching that is used in nursing education must be one that promotes the attainment of those goals.

THE NEED FOR CONCEPTUAL CLARITY

A critical aspect in this process is determining how concepts will be presented in the curriculum—in other words, what will constitute a "conceptually adequate" approach for the purposes of the educational setting. Identifying concepts that are essential to the discipline and then providing students with a list of essential attributes, thus invoking the idea of "necessary and sufficient conditions" or an unchanging set of attributes is not consistent with the ideology just described. This approach gives students the impression that concepts are static and perfectly clear, with distinguishable boundaries and with consistency regardless of context or situation. This approach promotes memorization rather than application, because students undoubtedly will be focused on learning the essential attributes so those can be recited at a later time (for example, on multiple choice tests). This approach also fails to acknowledge the critical and essential processes of application and also of conceptual change.

What is needed for teaching purposes (and for concept development in general) is a way to identify and communicate some of the important core features of a concept while allowing for other considerations such as application, variation across contexts, conceptual change, and the fact that concepts are never perfect or fully finished products, nor are they always perfectly distinct from each other. These observations about concepts do not mean our concepts have serious problems; rather, it is important to recognize these grey areas to enable the growth and change that is essential to dynamic application and that allow for variations across cultures, contexts, and individuals. It is the more rigid approach that actually possesses far greater shortcomings, even though the illusion of clarity and exactness may be comforting to student and instructor alike. Most students seem to strive for some sort of absolute answer to what *Dignity* really is, once and for all, or what constitutes a *Person*. Even a concept such as *Illness* would be received well with some sort of absolute answer. Yet all of these concepts must be amenable to variation across individuals, cultures, contexts, and the variation required by new discoveries. As with all concepts, both *Dignity* and *Illness* have needed to change as society has changed and as new research forced reconsideration and further development of these concepts.

Procedures for Concept Analysis and Clarification

The process of identifying the core components of a concept is concept clarification, which most commonly is accomplished by using methods of concept analysis. Concept analysis is not an end point—analyze the concept and be done with it. Instead, it should be viewed as a useful step in a larger process of concept development. Various forms of inquiry, such as traditional scientific work, all contribute to knowledge related to the concepts being studied. Research of many types helps to clarify and expand knowledge about the subject being studied. On one level, this is all part

BOX 3.2 ■ Approaches to Concept Analysis Used in Nursing

Morse (1995)—Principle-Based Concept Analysis
Norris (1982)—Concept Clarification
Walker and Avant (1983, 2011)—Concept Analysis
Rodgers (1989, 2000)—Evolutionary Cycle of Concept Development
Schwartz-Barcott and Kim (1986)—Hybrid Model of Concept Development

of the process of concept development, not merely the generation of new information or "facts." Theory development also requires attention to concepts, and often the process of concept development is a major focus of expanding and clarifying an existing theory. Keeping concept analysis within the broader context of concept development will help students remember that concepts are not static and that they, too, can continue to develop their own concepts as they apply and evaluate their own conceptual knowledge. The analysis of concepts is a beneficial and often a critical starting point in this process.

Concept analysis is well established in the literature of nursing, and several different methodologies exist for this purpose. Box 3.2 contains a list of some of the methodologies that have been used in nursing studies. Until recently, however, little information was available that would help researchers or others interested in this type of work identify and design a methodologically and philosophically sound approach. It is not uncommon in the literature to find that authors followed a particular approach because it was recommended by an instructor, it was found frequently in the literature, or it seemed easy to follow (Rodgers, 2000). Convenience and commonality, however, are not appropriate criteria for selecting a procedure for inquiry. Exploring concepts for purposes of concept-based teaching may not be formal research, but it still calls for rigorous and sound inquiry. Similarly, the process and the presentation of the concept need to be consistent with the philosophical approach to concepts that is represented throughout the curriculum. Many of the concepts of interest to faculty for inclusion in the curricula may have completed analyses available in the literature. However, many will not, and even some of those that do exist may present conflicting results. The key to faculty using the conceptual approach to teaching is to provide conceptual definitions that are clear, that make sense in application, and that are not so rigid and static as to stifle the students' thinking.

In selecting the approach to clarify a concept for purposes of concept-based teaching, the instructor also should consider the nature of the concept to be analyzed. Some concepts are suited to more specificity, such as those that are represented by diagnostic criteria or taxonomies. Concepts that are newer may fit this category also as they typically do not evidence a long history of conceptual change. It also may be possible to identify physical or tangible objects that serve as examples of such concepts, which can make clarification and description easier to accomplish, keeping in mind actual objects that represent the concept. An example of such a concept would be *Bacteria,* which has a specific, clear, and easily discernible definition. Physiological concepts, in general, will be amenable to more precision, whereas concepts pertaining to intangible qualities such as emotion, behavior, and social phenomena (the psychosocial concepts) are going to show more variation and vagueness. Morse, Mitcham, Hupcey, and Tason (1996) referred to some concepts as being "mature" in reference to the length of their existence and presumed state of development. It is often assumed that more mature concepts are capable of greater precision because of their longevity. However, a lengthy period of use only exposes a concept to more change and variation, and sometimes to radical change. Although the history of the emergence and evolution of a concept can shed a great deal of light on its definition and use over time, it is not an essential consideration in deciding how to proceed with concept development.

EVOLUTIONARY APPROACH TO CONCEPT DEVELOPMENT

For the purposes of concept-based teaching, especially instilling in students an appreciation for conceptual change over time, the approach to concept clarification based on the Evolutionary View of Concept Development (Rodgers, 2000) is very useful and consistent with contemporary philosophical views of concepts. In this view, clarification of a concept serves as an important step in a broader process of concept development. It is desirable that students not only understand important concepts but that they see their application of concepts as feeding back into the developmental process. Analysis is the starting point in an ongoing cycle of concept development.

Therefore concept analysis is the process of breaking a concept down to identify the attributes that constitute its definition. It also involves identifying other aspects of the concept, particularly contextual factors, that are important in being able to use the concept effectively. Because concepts have an important "use," it is possible to look at how it is used to determine what makes up the concept. For the purposes of concept-based teaching, the most likely sources of data for examining the use of the concept will be the professional literature, such as publications in nursing and related journals. Concepts also are expressed in other forms, such as through spoken language and even through the performing arts, and beneficial teaching strategies can be created that involve the arts in some form. In most cases, however, the appropriate starting point is the professional literature. For some concepts, it also can be illuminating to examine popular constructions of a concept, particularly for those that can have a strong individual interpretation or cultural and contextual variation. The concept of *Grief*, for example, not only has a large base of professional literature but can be found in a wide array of popular literature as well. Understanding these perspectives, as expressed by people experiencing the concept, can provide important insights to help the student apply the concept and understand variations in the concept across settings and situations.

Using the Evolutionary View of Concepts for Teaching

The Evolutionary View is associated with a formal process of concept analysis that can be used in a thorough attempt at concept clarification for the purposes of teaching. This approach looks similar to the one advocated by the popular writings of Walker and Avant (2011). In fact, all approaches to concept analysis have a great deal in common with regard to the specific activities that are conducted as part of the analysis. There are, however, what may seem subtle but actually are quite profound differences.

The Evolutionary View is not a variant of approaches based on the work of Wilson (1963), such as that proposed by Walker and Avant. For purposes of developing clear concepts for concept-based teaching, the process identified in the following sections can be very effective. Note that it also can be used in teaching, taking students through the process of the analysis to ensure that all of the components of the concept are presented clearly through the learning experience. For a thorough discussion of this approach, please see the description provided elsewhere (Rodgers, 2000). A simplified version, intended for ease of use by instructors and faculty, is provided here.

MISCONCEPTIONS AND CLARIFICATIONS

Misconception: The various approaches to concept analysis found in the literature are essentially the same.

Clarification: The various approaches to concept analysis appear similar in many ways, but the differences actually are quite profound.

IDENTIFYING THE CONCEPT OF INTEREST

First, it is essential to identify the concept of interest. The emphasis needs to be on the idea that is communicated, not the word that is used to discuss it. Words are expressions of ideas, not the ideas themselves. Using the example of *Grief* again, the instructor needs to determine what term best expresses the concept to be discussed. Some obvious possibilities include the terms "bereavement" and "loss". *Grief* also might be discussed in the context of stress, coping, adaptation, resilience, and other terms that express related ideas. It is important to be clear about what the concept of interest is and then what term is best used to express that concept. The selection of the term will guide the clarification process, along with any teaching and learning interactions with students. As the example of grief indicates, there may be two terms that seem to express similar ideas, and it may be appropriate to explore both to determine which term is most appropriate and has the broadest support. The terms "grief" and "bereavement" both have relevance in the exploration of the same concept, although a thorough review of the literature does reveal some differences (Rodgers & Cowles, 2000).

Another example of a situation in which the selection of the concept and associated terminology is critical to conceptual understanding is the concept of *Adherence*, also referred to using the term "compliance" (Bissonnette, 2017). Conceptually, the argument has been made that *Compliance* is quite different from *Adherence*, with the term adherence used to diminish what many viewed as the "more paternalistic" (p. 46) approach associated with "compliance." This is an example of why it is important to focus on the concept, or the thinking that goes on, and not the word. It is possible that either term is learned by students as essentially the same thing. It also is possible that the two terms conjure very different ideas. For teaching in this area, it is important to explore the changes in terminology, acknowledging the controversy and contrasts, to help students acquire a stronger grasp of this concept. This also serves as a good example of how the selection of terminology is important in identifying examples of the concept as a literature search for "compliance" may not reveal the very closely related literature of "adherence" and that the focus on thinking—the idea or concept—is the critical element in learning.

DETERMINE THE RELEVANT CONTEXT

The process of concept clarification and development requires attention to the context of the use of the concept. The concept of *Compliance* or *Adherence* may be different in health care than it is in an engineering application. A more obvious example is the concept of *coping*. In a health care context, *coping* refers to behavioral and cognitive means of adjusting to various situations. *Coping*, as a concept, involves not only a positive outcome, as in, "She is coping well with her new challenges," but the process of making responses to changing stimuli. *Coping* often is discussed in health care in the context of other concepts such as *Stress, Adaptation*, and *Resilience* (Giddens, 2017). The term "coping" also can be found in regard to woodworking, such as "coping saw"(Walker & Avant, 2011). In some respects, this concept is similar, because the saw makes precise and fine adjustments to produce intricate patterns in the material being cut. The saw makes it possible for wood, for example, to respond to its surroundings to make a precise fit. Walker and Avant (2011) also identify "coping" in reference to a type of garment and refer to all of these examples as varied uses of the same concept, arguing that all of the examples should be included in the analysis. This approach would be misleading on a number of levels, however, because these uses and ideas of coping clearly miss the intricacies and important aspects of coping as a psychological and cognitive process (Giddens, 2017; Rodgers, 2000). Furthermore, this approach is a solid example of confusing terminology, or the use of a word, with the use of a concept. Keeping the focus on the concept of *Coping* that, for nursing purposes, is used and discussed in regard to a distinct type of human experience, will help students focus and ensure a clear emphasis on the concept of interest rather than on the terminology. Settings and application also may include considerations about age, culture, and care context, to the extent that those considerations are relevant. These applications are just a few in a long list of possible applications that exist for many concepts of interest in nursing.

It is important at this stage to point out that even though the activities are enumerated here, thus giving the impression that they occur in sequential fashion, the process of concept clarification is not a linear process at all. Each activity discussed can be affected by all of the others; for example, determining what terminology will work best for a literature review will be affected by the literature that is uncovered during the review. This terminology may again need to be changed as literature is reviewed. It is important to see the flow of activities as an iterative process, with each activity influenced by the others.

COLLECT DATA TO CLARIFY THE CONCEPT

Data collection proceeds once some of the critical decisions about the concept have been made, at least on a preliminary basis. As previously noted, data collection may lead the faculty to look at other terminology, sources, or contexts. Consequently, even though data collection is a major focus of the analysis and development processes, it is not an isolated endeavor that is pursued without regard for the other parts of the process. For concept-based teaching, data collection will be focused on collecting sufficient information to determine the major components of the concept. These components include the attributes of the concept—in other words, its key components—along with discussion of the context in which the concept is used. Context can include social and cultural considerations in addition to elements that reflect a time sequence. Situations or events that occur before an instance of the concept and those that occur after are typically discussed as "antecedents" and "consequences," respectively. For purposes of concept-based teaching, these situations or events might be more appropriately discussed in a general time sequence as precursors or "causes," if appropriate, or other terminology consistent with a clinical application, and consequences can be discussed as outcomes or sequelae or simply as consequences. Antecedents and consequences help to put the concept in an application setting so that students can understand not just the concept but when they might see examples of it and what creates a situation in which the concept is applicable, along with possible outcomes. Data that help answer these questions are derived from the literature and then are analyzed to develop clear indicators of the effective use of the concept. Proceeding in this manner reveals the "state of the science" regarding the concept for nursing application (Rodgers, 2000).

IDENTIFY EXEMPLARS

Finally, exemplars of the proper use of the concept help students grasp the application of the concept in the appropriate context and make the concept come to life. Exemplars, in this view, are not the same as "model cases." A model case, according to Wilson (1963), is a case "which we are absolutely sure" is an instance of the concept in that it contains all of the conditions that are necessary and sufficient" to comprise an example of the concept (p. 28). Walker and Avant (2011) include these and other types of cases in their approach to analysis. There is a significant problem with "model" cases, however, in that they may give the impression of greater clarity and certainty than is appropriate. The term "exemplar" is used purposefully in the Evolutionary Method to reflect the fact that these examples ideally can be found in "real life" and are not models or paradigmatic cases that are constructed by the person doing the analysis (Fehr, 1988; Rodgers, 2000). Multiple examples can be used to show the nuances of the concept in different applications and contexts and to help students accept how boundaries more often are fuzzy and unclear than distinct and rigid. Exemplars that show changes over time and the influence of new research can be an important part of nursing socialization and help students gain an appreciation for evidence-based practice and how the evidence often is changing. Concepts related to sleep, for example, have changed considerably in recent years as sleep has become an established specialty area and as knowledge has changed about the importance of sleep and various disruptors. The concept of *Sleep* can be discussed in the context of differentiation from fatigue, as a factor in metabolic regularity, in relation to sleep-disordered breathing, and in association with cognitive functioning, to name just a few examples of how sleep is of concern. As another example, the concept of *Infection* is one that nurses work with frequently, and it may be discussed with regard to a patient who has an infectious process and with regard to primary prevention. As part of this process, it may be beneficial to point out where there is a need for further knowledge development or research and where vague areas and questions remain regarding the concept. The more that students can be helped to see how knowledge constantly changes and to view all sides of a concept and a wide array of applications, the more they are likely to be able to think critically and creatively and solve problems in actual clinical application.

It is not necessary to pursue this in-depth process of concept clarification for every concept addressed in the curriculum. It would be prohibitive to do a formal analysis, using a rigorous sample drawn from the literature, for every concept that will be discussed. Fortunately, references and textbooks exist that present some of the work that has been done along these lines. In addition, a literature search will uncover an extensive number of articles presenting the results of analyses although, as with all research, the quality of the studies vary. For concepts that are particularly confusing or vague or the focal point of disagreement among the faculty, a formal analysis may be of benefit. Even if a formal analysis is not completed, however, the faculty need to be comfortable presenting the key elements of the concept and can structure the presentation according to the aspects of the concept that are essential for understanding.

Bringing the Concept Presentation to Life

The results of concept analysis, when reported in the literature, may seem very tedious or cumbersome to read. There typically is a listing of each of the major components with varying amounts of discussion about each component. For purposes of inquiry, where it is necessary to be clear about the status of each component of the concept to identify directions for future development, this information may be useful. For education, however, it is more important that the concept be presented in a way that comes alive for students. The necessary degree of conceptual clarity must be present, but the analysis and presentation will be more effective if the components are woven together in a manner that helps students grasp the appearance and use of the concept in real-life situations.

The intent of concept clarification activities in a concept-based curriculum is to help the students grasp the concept and be able to use it effectively. This includes giving students sufficient information to (1) recognize the occurrence of the concept and be clear and appropriate in its application; (2) value the contextual elements; (3) recognize and use associated terminology; (4) explore distinctions among similar concepts; and (5) appreciate the nuances and subtleties of the concept and its areas of imperfection. There is no limit to how a concept can be presented to help students grasp these components. Whatever the focus of discussion, however, there must be a "conceptually adequate" definition that demonstrates the prevailing attributes of the concept and its scope of application.

Case studies can be an important strategy to help students grasp the concept, but it is important not to fall into the trap of "model cases." Model cases, as noted previously, can place inappropriate boundaries on a concept and cause the individual learning the concept to assume too narrow a scope of application. The learner may reach the conclusion that, if such an example is a model, then *all* instances of the concept will appear to be similar. Even relatively clear-cut concepts, such as *Mobility*, have numerous variations related to arthritis, postoperative ambulation, amputation, and many more instances, in addition to the positive aspects such as athleticism. Focusing on a model case of *Mobility*, perhaps in the case of a distance runner who clearly is very "mobile," will present an unnecessary and unrealistic example that does not show the range of use of the concept and its relevance in numerous instances in nursing. Another example is *Asepsis*, which is closely related to the concepts of *Sepsis* and *Infection*, either of which can be found along a continuum ranging from simple, localized infection to systemic septic shock and intractable conditions. Exemplars, presented from a variety of perspectives and showing the concept in numerous contexts, will help students grasp not only the defining characteristics of the concept but the many ways in which it can be used appropriately.

Summary

Methods of concept development, particularly concept analysis and clarification, are essential in a concept-based curriculum. Following a documented approach to clarification can help ensure that the appropriate components of a concept are understood well, presented clearly, and described in relevant contexts similar to how students are expected to use the concepts. Essential components of a concept, which are sufficient to provide a high degree of clarity, can be articulated within a concept development framework. This can provide a structure for presentation and discussion, as well as for making sure that all critical aspects are addressed. It is important, however, that the approach to analysis and clarification be one that promotes critical thinking, relevant application, and a strong grasp of the concept as demonstrated by the students' ability to use the concept effectively (Rodgers, 2000). Presenting concepts from a philosophical perspective that acknowledges conceptual change and helps students actively engage in that process through evaluation of the usefulness and effectiveness of concepts can promote not only concept learning but the spirit of inquiry, adaptability, and ongoing evaluation that is essential to effective nursing practice and growth.

References

Bissonnette JB. Adherence. In: Giddens JF, ed. *Concepts for Nursing Practice*. 2nd ed. St. Louis, MO: Mosby; 2017:46–53.

Fehr B. Prototype analysis of the concepts of love and commitment. *J Pers Soc Psychol*. 1988;55:557–579.

Giddens JF. Coping. In: Giddens JF, ed. *Concepts for Nursing Practice*. 2nd ed. St. Louis, MO: Mosby; 2017:309–316.

Morse JM, Mitcham C, Hupcey JE, Tason MC. Criteria for concept evaluation. *J Adv Nurs*. 1996;24:385–390.

Morse JM. Exploring the theoretical basis of nursing knowledge using advanced techniques of concept analysis. *Adv Nurs Sci*. 1995;17:31–46.

Norris CM. *Concept Clarification in Nursing*. Rockville, MD: Aspen; 1982.

Oxford Dictionary of English. 2nd ed. Oxford, United Kingdom: Oxford University; 2005.

Rodgers BL, Cowles KV. The concept of grief: an evolutionary perspective. In: Rodgers BL, Knafl KA, eds. *Concept Development in Nursing: Foundations, Techniques, and Applications*. 2nd ed. Philadelphia, PA: WB Saunders; 2000:103–117.

Rodgers BL. Concept analysis: an evolutionary view. In: Rodgers BL, Knafl KA, eds. *Adv Nurs Sci*. 2nd ed. Philadelphia, PA: WB Saunders; 2000:77–102.

Rodgers BL. Concepts, analysis, and the development of nursing knowledge: the evolutionary cycle. *J Adv Nurs*. 1989;14:330–335.

Schwartz-Barcott D, Kim HS. A hybrid model for concept development. In: Chinn PL, ed. *Nursing Research Methodology: Issues and Implementation*. Rockville, MD: Aspen; 1986:91–101.

Walker LO, Avant KC. *Strategies for Theory Construction in Nursing*. Norwalk, CT: Appleton-Century-Crofts; 1983.

Walker LO, Avant KC. *Strategies for Theory Construction in Nursing*. 5th ed. Upper Saddle River, NJ: Pearson Education; 2011.
Wilson J. *Thinking with Concepts*. London, United Kingdom: Cambridge University Press; 1963.

CHAPTER 4

Developing a Concept-Based Curriculum

Jean Giddens

Curriculum development, regardless of the discipline, the type of learning program, or the level of learner, follows a general and predictable process. In academic institutions, faculty members are responsible for the development, implementation, and evaluation of the curriculum. A curriculum should reflect and support the overarching goals of the academic institution and nursing school. Nurse educators must also consider changes in professional nursing standards, health care trends, higher education, and the general society when undertaking curriculum work. Special interest groups, stakeholders, and a number of policy, regulatory, and political variables must also be addressed. Needless to say, curriculum work is a complex process that requires many resources. Several books have been written that describe curriculum development and revision in detail; such detail is beyond the scope of this chapter. The intent of this chapter is to provide a general overview of curriculum development as a frame of reference and then focus on unique elements associated with curriculum development when a conceptual approach is planned.

Overview of the Curriculum Development Process

The term *curriculum* refers to the arrangement of content within courses that form an academic program. The purpose of a curriculum is to provide an organizational structure to the content within an academic program so that learners can successfully achieve predetermined outcomes. In many cases, nursing schools or departments offer multiple programs (or concentrations within a program), thus multiple curricular plans are used—one to support each program and concentration.

Curriculum work is not a one-time event but rather a continuous process. As Fig. 4.1 shows, a new curriculum or a curriculum revision occurs based on evidence that changes must be made. After a curriculum is developed or revised, faculty and institutional approval must be gained before it is implemented. Implementation of the curriculum occurs with a clearly identified plan to evaluate program learning outcomes and assess student learning. Data are regularly collected and analyzed by faculty, which in turn provides evidence for curriculum changes as they are needed.

INTERNAL AND EXTERNAL CONTEXT FOR CURRICULUM CHANGE

It is often said that faculty "own" the curriculum, meaning that faculty are accountable for continually developing, implementing, evaluating, and revising the curriculum. Several internal and external forces and issues play a significant role in the curriculum; thus nurse educators must maintain an ongoing awareness of these contextual factors. Internal factors include expertise of the faculty in curriculum development, other curricula offered by a nursing school or department, institutional policies, institutional culture, student characteristics, physical resources, and human resources (e.g., the number of faculty, staff, and students enrolled). Professional practice standards,

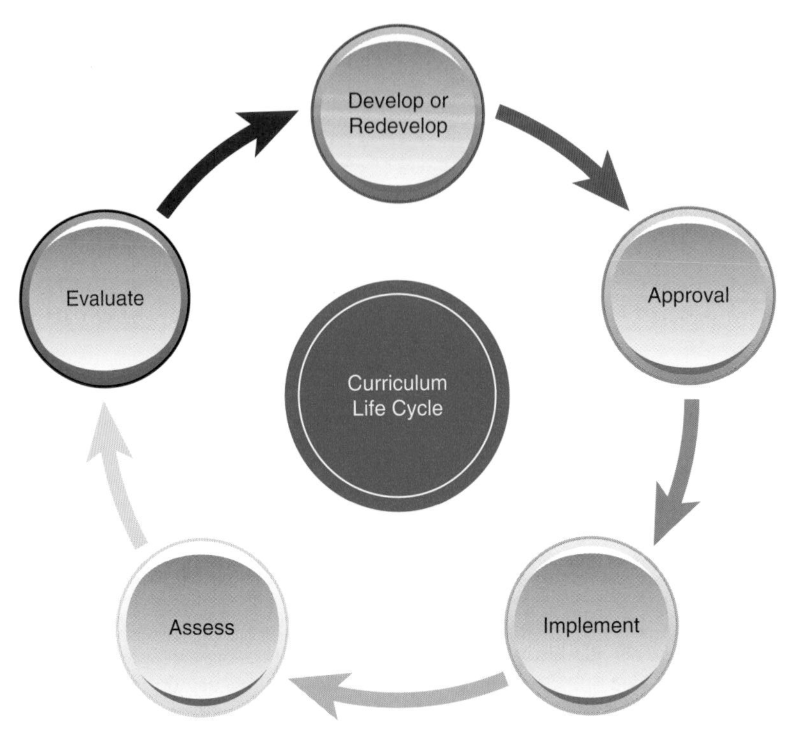

Fig. 4.1 The life cycle of a curriculum.

accreditation standards, regulatory bodies, and clinical agencies are examples of external drivers of change that have policy implications. Other important external factors that have influenced curriculum change in nursing include seminal position statements and reports (such as *The Future of Nursing* [IOM, 2010], *Educating Nurses: A Radical Call for Transformation* (Benner et al., 2010); competencies (such as Quality and Safety Education in Nursing [QSEN] competencies [QSEN, n.d.) and Interprofessional Education Collaboration [IPEC] competencies [IPEC, 2011]; and the rise of technologies for simulation and online learning. Characteristics of the community served (such as population demographics and culture), socioeconomic factors, health care access, and employer demand represent other important external factors that are considered when designing or revising a curriculum.

MISSION, VISION, AND VALUES

As a starting point for curriculum development, faculty should consider the institutional mission and vision statements of the parent institution, as well as those stated by the nursing school or department. A mission statement explains organizational purpose or meaning; better stated, the mission statement describes why an entity exists. A vision is a statement of what an entity wants to be or what it wishes to accomplish. Thus mission and vision statements serve as a compass for the parent institution, as well as the nursing school or department. Consistency and clear linkages between the nursing school mission and vision and the institutional mission and vision statements are required (Fig. 4.2).

A school's philosophy is a statement of values or beliefs held collectively by the faculty, providing consistency and integrity to all curriculum elements (Csokasy, 2002). These values and

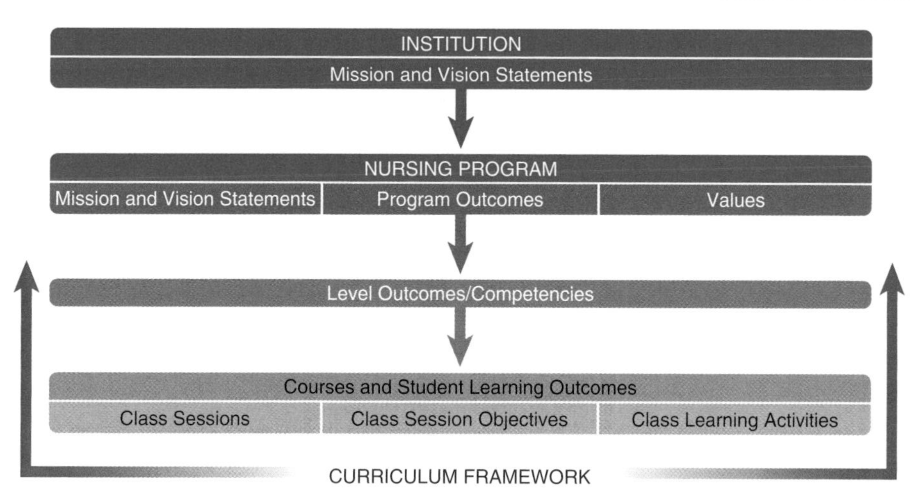

Fig. 4.2 Elements associated with a curriculum.

beliefs guide faculty in actions and decision-making related to curriculum and academic delivery. Developing a philosophical statement can be very time consuming and difficult. As a result, many schools have moved away from developing formal philosophical statements and have instead opted for core values for all members of the school. As this movement has occurred, a greater emphasis has been placed on having a well–thought-out organizational framework.

LEARNING OUTCOMES AND COMPETENCIES

Another central element of curriculum development is identification of learning outcomes. The term "outcome" refers to the end result of a process. A learning outcome is a specific statement that describes what a student will be able to do in a measurable way at a specified point in time. In many nursing programs, competencies are also incorporated into the curriculum. A competency is a general statement that describes the knowledge, skills, attitudes, and behaviors necessary for students to successfully perform in a professional context. Multiple competencies typically link to broad outcomes (Sullivan, 2016).

During the past 15 years, there has been growing trend in higher education for increased emphasis on learning outcomes and competencies as a result of completing an academic program. Curriculum goals and learning outcomes are not new, but the expectation of being able to measure and track students' accomplishment of learning outcomes certainly has increased with the assessment movement. This increased emphasis on learning outcomes is higher education's response to the public's expectation for accountability (Boland, 2004). The need to track learning outcomes, coupled with advancements in technology, has resulted in the development of applications specifically designed for outcome measurement and tracking of student learning outcomes.

There are different levels of learning outcomes and competencies. Program learning outcomes (also referred to as *end-of-program outcomes*) and program competencies are the "terminal" or "end points" that serve as the expected characteristics of graduates as a result of completing the program (Whittmann-Price and Fasolka, 2010). As a matter of sequence, faculty should consider identifying the program outcomes (and competencies, if applicable) after addressing the mission, vision, and philosophy and before identifying the organizational framework.

In addition to program learning outcomes, there is a need for "markers" at specified points within the curriculum to assess students' progress while in a program. These markers, known as "level learning outcomes" are statements of what is expected of students within three domains (cognitive, psychomotor, or affective). Likewise, when competencies are used, they are often described in terms of what the student should be able to do at specified points in the curriculum and often reflect skills that requires development over time. Learning outcomes and competency statements drive assessment of student learning within the curriculum and thus serve as the structural foundation of program evaluation. For this reason, it is critical these components link clearly throughout the curriculum.

CURRICULUM DESIGN: DEVELOPING AN ORGANIZATIONAL FRAMEWORK

An organizational framework is essentially the blueprint or design of a curriculum, helping to clarify the scope of content and how it will fit together. It provides a mental picture of how the curricular elements interface with the curriculum approach. The process of developing the organizational framework includes identifying and defining the structural elements (e.g., themes, principles, threads, competencies, or concepts) to gain a shared understanding about what these elements mean. In addition, developing a clear vision and message about how the curriculum elements link together is critical. These elements must be constructed so that program learning outcomes and competencies are achievable.

COURSE DESIGN

Courses within a curriculum should reflect the program learning outcomes and level competencies. In other words, individual courses within a curriculum should be logically structured to facilitate students' achievement of the level learning outcomes and competencies that support program learning outcomes and competencies. For this reason, level competencies are used as a basis for course development.

Expectations of student learning within courses are written as course learning outcomes (or in some cases, course competencies). Course learning outcomes are more specific and concrete than level outcomes; these outcomes not only provide the foundation for course development but also for assessment of student learning within the course. Clear linkages between course learning outcomes and level learning outcomes (or competencies) help to ensure curricular cohesion; in a concept-based curriculum, the outcomes should link to concepts. Student learning outcomes and competencies have gradually replaced the behavioral objectives approach historically used in higher education. An ongoing debate about the use of objectives, student learning outcomes, and competencies has been reflected in the nursing education literature for more than a decade (Bastable, 2013; Caputi, 2010; Goudreau et al., 2009; Nelson, Howell, Larson, & Karpiuk, 2001; Whittmann-Price & Fasolka, 2010). Regardless of the decisions made by a faculty to use student learning outcomes, competencies, or objectives at the course level, the most important point is that they provide clarity about the content focus and expectations of students.

The development of the course takes shape by developing a syllabus. Specific elements for course development include determining the type of course (e.g., lab, clinical, seminar, or didactic), the course description, student learning outcomes for the course, the number of academic credits, course delivery, a course outline (i.e., delineation of specific topics/content featured within the course), and planned strategies for teaching, learning, and evaluation. Teaching, learning, and evaluation strategies should align with the student learning outcomes and the type of course. Arrangement and sequencing of the courses collectively should be considered to ensure continuity, consistency, and balance. Such a process occurs regardless of type of curriculum design.

CURRICULUM MODEL

A visual model of the curricular framework shows the association between the concepts and elements within the curriculum. This can help faculty and students to gain a better understanding the curriculum. Boland advises a "less-is-more" principle related to the development of curricular models, warning that too complex of a model leads faculty to "spend more time trying to interpret and understand the framework than they do actually implementing and evaluating it" (Boland, 2012, p. 144).

PROGRAM EVALUATION

Evaluation is an organized and ongoing appraisal of the curriculum to determine strengths and weaknesses. It should include all curriculum elements and professional standards, as well as the success of the students and graduates of the program. Program evaluation is planned as a part of curriculum development, and continues during and after implementation. A strong evaluation plan involves having a clear understanding of the evaluation standards and type of data to collect, a consistent data collection process, and a clear plan for data analysis. Curricular improvements should be data driven as a result of this process.

As mentioned previously, program learning outcomes, competencies, and student learning outcomes at the course level provide the infrastructure for an evaluation plan. Data should be collected at the course level, at markers along the way, and at the end of the program using a variety of data collection methods. Data sources can include students, faculty, employers, preceptors, nurses, and curriculum and course documents.

Developing a Curriculum Using the Conceptual Approach

Educators interested in developing a concept-based curriculum follow a similar process described in the previous section. This section will take each of the steps and describe in greater detail unique elements when developing a curriculum using a conceptual approach.

INTERNAL AND EXTERNAL CONTEXT FOR CURRICULUM CHANGE

The same contextual factors previously described apply to a concept-based curriculum and there are a few other factors to be aware of. One of the most important internal contexts to consider is faculty expertise related to the conceptual approach. Expertise is needed for appropriate decision-making and to clearly articulate the conceptual approach to administrators, other faculty, students, and external stakeholders. This expertise is also needed to address resistance.

External factors especially important to consider when adopting a conceptual approach are the perspectives of the employers and nurses within the community. It is essential that this group of stakeholders understand why the curriculum is changing and how it is envisioned; eliciting their support and input is critical. Most employers welcome a change in the education system, especially if it means that the nursing graduates will have higher-level thinking and problem-solving skills. Communicating the competencies of graduates is important for prospective employers. Nurses in the community, particularly those who interface directly or indirectly with students, must have an understanding of the changes that will occur, especially with regard to clinical education. Most nurses welcome a change in the educational system if it means that clinical education is less burdensome to the practice areas and if their input is solicited.

MISSION, VISION, AND VALUES

Faculty adopting a concept-based curriculum should consider the institutional mission and vision statements of the parent institution as well as those stated by the nursing school or department—an expectation consistent with any curriculum development process. It is possible that the conceptual approach will influence a revision of the nursing school's mission, vision, or philosophy statement, although it is also possible these statements can remain unchanged.

LEARNING OUTCOMES AND COMPETENCIES

After the mission and vision have been considered, curriculum committees usually develop or revise the program learning outcomes (end of program learning outcomes) and competencies (as applicable). Program learning outcomes are sequenced before the curriculum design because the these serve as a beacon or directional endpoint. Faculty often ask how the program learning outcomes should be stated for a concept-based curriculum. The curriculum design is essentially a blueprint of the curriculum and is driven by the mission, vision, and program learning outcomes; in other words, it is not the program learning outcomes that are different, but rather the way the curriculum is packaged. For example, a common program learning outcome of an undergraduate curriculum may read something like this: *Collaborate as a member of an interdisciplinary team to improve the quality of health care.*

Such an outcome is a desired expectation of any nursing graduate from any nursing program regardless of the type of curricular design of the nursing program. However, the curricular design is the vehicle faculty choose to ensure that students can achieve this learning outcome. Thus, there is little difference in this process, although the design should be taken into account to ensure that the structure fits the identified learning outcomes and competencies. Competencies are often used in concept-based curricula to assess what a student knows and can do at designated points of the curriculum. In a concept-based curriculum, competencies should clearly link to the program learning outcomes and concepts within the curriculum (Table 4.1).

TABLE 4.1 ■ **Linkages Between Program Learning Outcomes, Concepts, Competencies, and Course Learning Outcomes in a Concept-Based Curriculum**

Curricular Element	Example
Program learning outcome	Collaborate as a member of an interdisciplinary team to improve the quality of health care.
Curriculum Concepts	• Health Care Quality • Safety • Collaboration
Level Competencies	**Semester 1:** Assesses own understanding of collaboration to determine strength and weaknesses as an effective member of a health care team. **Semester 2:** Appraises the effectiveness and appropriateness of collaboration among members of the health care team in patient care delivery. **Semester 3:** Incorporates the concepts of quality, safety, and collaboration into clinical experiences as a member of health care teams. **Semester 4:** Effectively participates as a member of an interprofessional team to deliver safe and quality care.
Examples of course learning outcomes from two Professional Nursing Concepts courses.	**NURS 317**: Describe the concepts of Health Care Quality, Safety, and Collaboration and influences on health care delivery. **NURS 441**: Analyze the concepts of Health Care Quality, Safety, and Collaboration as foundational elements to effective health care delivery.

MISCONCEPTIONS AND CLARIFICATIONS

Misconception: The program learning outcomes are written completely differently when developing a concept-based curriculum—focusing only on concepts.

Clarification: Program learning outcomes reflect what a student can do as a result of the program and are written similar to program learning outcomes of traditional curricular design. Curricular concepts should link to program learning outcomes.

DEVELOPING A DESIGN FOR A CONCEPT-BASED CURRICULUM

One of the truly unique hallmarks of developing a concept-based curriculum is with the design. As mentioned previously, curriculum design is an organizational framework—or better stated, the blueprint for the curriculum. This process includes selecting and defining the concepts and determining how the concepts will be linked together within the curriculum. Fig. 4.3 shows these general steps.

Concept Categories

Once the decision to adopt a concept-based curriculum is made, there is a tendency for faculty to immediately begin identifying and negotiating concepts to be included. However, a step that ideally precedes this process is the identification and development of concept categories. Concept categories provide structure to the curriculum through the organization of concepts and provide greater clarity about what the concepts represent. Development of the concept category involves establishing criteria or parameters regarding how concepts for each category are selected, identified, and applied. Parameters establish the rules or criteria involved in determining whether a concept fits within a category and also provide some guidelines regarding how it is framed and eventually taught. For example, concept categories might be related to patient populations, areas of health care practice, or even philosophical perspectives about health. If a large number of concepts fit within a broad category, subcategories (or macroconcepts) are useful for further organization. The number and type of concept categories used within a curriculum can vary considerably and is one of the ways a curriculum from one school can distinguish itself from another. Three common concept categories are presented and described as examples in the following sections.

Health and Illness Concepts. Health and illness concepts represent a patient's health status in relationship to three general goals of health care: the promotion of health, the prevention of disease, and the treatment of illness. These goals are interrelated and often thought of in terms of functional processes. An established categorical description used to determine whether a concept fits in the

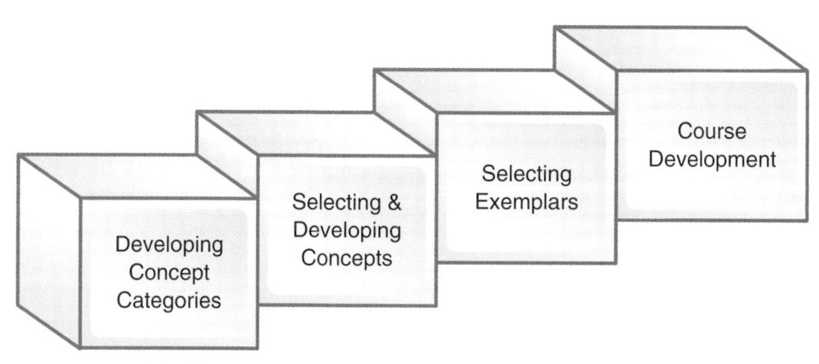

Fig. 4.3 Critical steps for concept-based curriculum design.

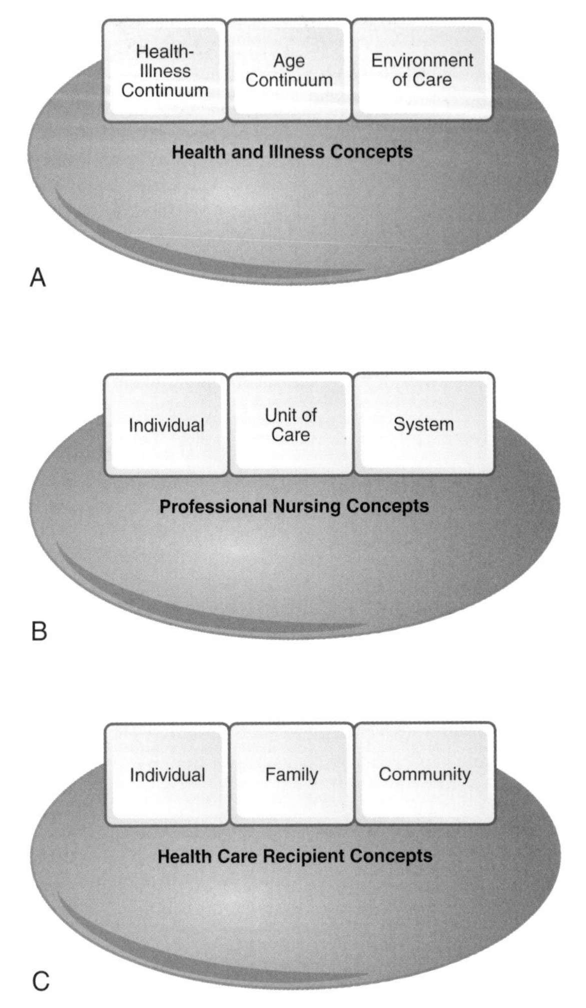

Fig. 4.4 Concept categories and parameters. **A,** Health and illness concepts. **B,** Professional nursing concepts. **C,** Health care recipient concepts.

category might be something as simple as "*A physiological or psychosocial health response*." Concepts such as *Gas Exchange*, *Infection*, *Mobility*, *Immunity*, *Cognition*, and *Mood* clearly fit, whereas concepts such as *Delegation*, *Policy*, and *Ethics* clearly do not. Health and illness concepts are considered from three contexts: *health continuum*, *life span continuum*, and *environment of care*. These contexts serve as guiding principles related to how the concepts are selected, presented, and applied (Fig. 4.4).

For example, the concept *Immunity* represents conditions across the health-illness continuum (health promotion, acute illness, and chronic conditions) and across the life span continuum (infants, children, adolescents, adults, and older adults), and care delivery occurs across multiple environments (within hospital units and clinics, and from a community health perspective, public health perspective, and global perspective). Parameters such as these help with the selection process and provide clarity for use within the curriculum.

Because the health and illness concept category is very large, macroconcepts help to further organize concepts. For example, a curriculum committee may wish to use a macroconcept such as

Oxygenation and Homeostasis as a category for *Perfusion, Gas Exchange,* and *Clotting*. Likewise, the concepts *Infection, Mobility,* and *Tissue Integrity* logically fit under the macroconcept Protection and Movement (Table 4.2). Concepts organized within a macroconcept are closely interrelated.

Professional Nursing Concepts. Concepts that represent the critical attributes and collectively describe professional nursing practice are referred to as professional nursing concepts. These concepts are associated with professional comportment—or in other words, these concepts link with the identity of nursing as a health care profession. Many of these concepts actually link more broadly to desired behaviors of all health care providers. Concepts such as *Professionalism, Ethics, Collaboration,* and *Patient Education* all clearly fit in a category such as this.

Established parameters for the Professional Nursing Concept Category can be presented from the context of the *individual nurse*, the *unit of care*, and from a *system perspective* (see Fig. 4.4). For example, a concept such as *Policy* could be presented from the context of how policies affect a nurse in direct care (such as a uniform policy or a policy regarding central line care), how policies affect an organization (such as admission policies and reimbursement policies), and how policies affect the health care system. This concept could also be presented by taking one specific policy such as the Health Insurance Portability and Accountability Act and framing it from the context of the individual nurse, the organization, and the health care system.

Professional nursing concepts can be further organized with macroconcepts. For example, *Health Care Organizations, Health Care Economics, Health Policy,* and *Health Care Law* logically are grouped under the macroconcept *Health Care Infrastructure*. Likewise, the concepts *Care Coordination, Caregiving,* and *Palliative Care* logically fit under the macroconcept *Health Care Delivery* (Table 4.3).

TABLE 4.2 ■ **Examples of Macroconcepts and Concepts Within the Health and Illness Concept Category**

Concept Category	Macro-Concept	Concepts
Health and Illness Concepts	Oxygenation and Homeostasis	Perfusion, Gas Exchange, Clotting
	Protection and Movement	Immunity, Inflammation, Mobility, Tissue Integrity
	Regulation	Cellular Regulation, Thermoregulation, Glucose Regulation, Intracranial Regulation, Acid-Base Balance, Fluid and Electrolyte Balance, Nutrition, Elimination

TABLE 4.3 ■ **Examples of Macroconcepts and Concepts Within the Professional Nursing Concepts Category**

Concept Category	Macro-Concept	Concepts
Professional Nursing Concepts	Health Care Delivery	Care Coordination, Caregiving, Palliation
	Health Care Infrastructures	Health Care Organizations, Health Care Economics, Health Policy, Health Care Law
	Care Competencies	Communication, Collaboration, Health Care Quality, Safety, Technology, Informatics, Evidence
	Attributes and Roles	Professionalism, Clinical Judgment, Leadership, Ethics, Patient Education, Health Promotion

TABLE 4.4 ■ **Examples of Macroconcepts and Concepts Within the Health Care Recipient Category**

Concept Category	Macro-Concept	Concepts
Health Care Recipient	Attributes	Development, Functional Ability, Family Dynamics, Genetics
	Personal Preferences	Culture, Spirituality, Motivation, Adherence, Self-Management

BOX 4.1 ■ Hallmarks of Concepts for Nursing Education Curricula

- The concept represents an important group of conditions or situations (exemplars) encountered in nursing practice.
- The concept has application across multiple courses and contexts within the curriculum.
- The concept is useful to the learner.
- The concept can be used logically and consistently by all faculty.

Health Care Recipient Concepts. The health care delivery system has made major strides, particularly during the past two decades, to move from a disease-centered perspective (in which the health care providers controlled all aspects of care) to a patient-centered model whereby recipients of care are not only informed of care options but are partners in the care decisions. Delivery of patient-centered care requires the recognition that health care recipients are very diverse, and thus health care decisions must take into account the unique needs and preferences of the patient (IOM, 2001).

As a concept category, health care recipient concepts represent the unique and distinct attributes of all health care recipients. It is essential for nurses to understand these fundamental concepts for the successful delivery of patient-centered care. For organizational purposes, it may be useful to use the macroconcepts *Personal Preferences* and *Attributes and Resources* to further categorize concepts in this category (Table 4.4).

Health care recipient concepts are considered from three contexts: the *individual,* the *family,* and the *community* (with community care ranging from a local to a global perspective). These contexts serve as guiding principles related to how the concepts are selected, presented, and applied (see Fig. 4.4). For example, the concept *Culture* represents the shared attitudes, beliefs, traditions, norms, values, and preferences of individuals and groups of people. Culture should be considered when providing care to an individual health care recipient, and it should be considered in the context of that individual's family members—recognizing that there may be value conflict between the two. Culture from the perspective of community has applications for example, when doing work in public health nursing and when setting health policy. Context parameters such as these (the individual, the family, and the community) help with the selection process, and provide clarity for use within the curriculum.

Selecting and Identifying Concepts

Selecting concepts generally follows after or in conjunction with determining concept categories. Oftentimes, faculty will have ideas about certain concepts that should be included, and thus the formation of larger categories as concepts are discussed is natural. One of the biggest challenges, however, is determining how many and which concepts to include. The hallmarks of "good" or well-chosen concepts to include in a nursing curriculum are presented in Box 4.1. Typically, the concepts should be very familiar and understandable to nursing faculty because they represent the scope of nursing practice. If there is a lot of confusion among faculty about a proposed concept, it should be critically analyzed to determine if it represents a concept associated with a specialty (a microconcept) or if it really represents a larger category of concepts (a macroconcept). Distinctions between microconcepts and macroconcepts are presented in Chapter 1.

Because concepts should be reflective of contemporary nursing and health care practice, an examination of the nursing and other health sciences literature is helpful. Another strategy is to review the list of concepts included in other concept-based curricula. A study involving a survey of 10 nursing programs or consortiums using a concept-based curriculum identified a total of 54 benchmark concepts—in other words, those that were most prevalent among reporting schools (Table 4.5). This study validated that although most concept-based curricula have similar featured concepts, there is not a single "correct" list. In other words, one should expect some variability in the concepts if comparing concept-based curricula across a number of schools (Giddens, Wright, & Gray, 2012).

As concepts are recommended and negotiated, a consistent, systematic selection process should be applied to determine whether a concept is "accepted" or "rejected" for final inclusion in a curriculum. Five questions that link back to the hallmarks of a "good" concept can be used to facilitate such a process:

1. Does the concept represent an important group of conditions or situations (exemplars) encountered in nursing practice?
2. Can the concept be applied across multiple courses and contexts within the curriculum?
3. Is the concept useful to the learner? In other words, will the learner find a clear application of the concept to the courses and clinical experiences?
4. Can the concept be used logically and consistently by all faculty?
5. Is the concept sustainable? In other words, is this a concept that will be applicable in years to come?

Another element associated with concept selection is clearly defining and developing the concept. Faculty must have a shared understanding of the concept—how it is defined, what it represents, how it is applied, and how it will be taught. It is recommended that a template be followed so this work progresses consistently. The template may vary depending on the type of concept category, because one template does not necessarily work for all categories. A sample template for health and illness concepts and a template that works for professional nursing concept categories and health care recipient concepts are provided in Boxes 4.2 and 4.3, respectively.

TABLE 4.5 ■ **Common Concepts Used in Concept-Based Nursing Curricula**

Attribute Concepts	Professional Nursing Concepts	Health and Illness Concepts
Advocacy, Culture, Development, Diversity, Family, Spirituality	Caring, Clinical Judgment, Collaboration, Communication, Educator, Ethics, Evidence, Health Care Delivery, Economics, Law, Quality, Policy, Health Promotion, Leadership, Patent Centered, Professionalism, Safety, Technology, Informatics	Addiction, Anxiety, Cognition, Grief, Interpersonal Relationships, Mood, Self, Stress, Coping, Violence, Acid Base, Cellular Regulation, Behavior, Elimination, Fluid and Electrolyte, Gas Exchange, Immunity, Infection, Inflammation, Intracranial Regulation, Metabolism, Mobility, Nutrition, Pain/Comfort, Perfusion, Reproduction, Sensory Perception Sexuality, Sleep–Rest, Thermoregulation, Tissue Integrity

From Giddens J, Wright M, Gray I. Selecting concepts for a concept-based curriculum: application of a benchmark approach. *Journal of Nursing Education.* 2012;51(9):511-515.

BOX 4.2 ■ Sample Template for Health and Illness Concepts

- Definition
- Scope, type, or category(s)
- Individual risk factors and populations at risk
- Physiological process and consequences
- Assessment
- History
- Examination
- Diagnostic studies
- Clinical management
- Primary prevention
- Secondary prevention (screening)
- Collaborative interventions
- Interrelated concepts

BOX 4.3 ■ Sample Template for Professional Nursing Concepts and Health Care Recipient Concepts

- Definition
- Scope, type, or categories
- Attributes
- Theoretical links
- Context to nursing and health care
- Interrelated concepts

Selecting Exemplars

Exemplars provide clinical context for the concept. Exemplars—or "examples"—are necessary for deep conceptual learning because they provide a specific information, facts, topics and situations representing the concept for the broader, more abstract concept. Conceptual learning holds limited value unless students can anchor what they have learned to specific examples. From this perspective, this is where traditional nursing content fits in a concept-based curriculum. The use of facts and base information is absolutely necessary as part of the conceptual learning process because facts support conceptual learning, and conceptual understanding supports the students' ability to make generalizations—thus higher-order cognitive thinking. As an example, the student must understand facts associated with the heart and circulatory system as a foundation to learning the concept of perfusion. Furthermore, facts associated with exemplars (such as acute myocardial infarction) provide further opportunities to deepen the conceptual understanding associated with perfusion.

In a concept-based curriculum, exemplars are carefully selected to minimize excessive curricular content. It is not uncommon for nursing faculty to be initially skeptical about limiting the number of exemplars. The value of managing excessive curriculum content is based on the premise that when students gain a deep understanding of a concept, they are able to make connections from the concept to other exemplars—even ones they have not been formally taught in the classroom. It is also important to remember that students will be exposed to far more exemplars in the clinical setting when providing care to patients and families. Thus, an essential part of the concept-based curriculum is capitalizing on students' exposure to exemplars that are not formally taught in the didactic courses and helping students make purposeful cognitive connections.

Setting a process for exemplar selection helps to reduce the temptation to include exemplars that happen to be a favorite topic of one or more faculty, which tends to lead to a curriculum pitfall of excessive content. Ideally, data-driven decisions are made to select exemplars. When data driven decisions are made, students will be exposed to the most important and prevalent content. In other words, faculty will focus on the most common things the student will see in practice. Health and illness concepts are best selected on the basis of state, national, and global health incidence and prevalence statistics (such as the Centers for Disease Control and Prevention), although there may be an occasional situation where an exemplar is selected because it has unique value in illustrating the concept. Exemplars for professional nursing concepts and health care recipient attributes are best identified by current literature and contemporary events, although some events that are more historic may have particular value if they have forever influenced nursing and health care practice today.

Another challenge when selecting exemplars is that most exemplars link to multiple concepts; thus there is risk for duplication of content within the curriculum. For example, the exemplar pneumonia logically links to *Infection*, *Gas Exchange*, *Fatigue*, and *Fluid and Electrolyte Balance*—but it is completely unnecessary to teach it four times as an exemplar of four concepts! A curriculum plan or map should be developed that clearly shows exemplars used for each concept. When teaching a specific exemplar, the lesson plan should include time for students to reflect on concepts that are interrelated with the exemplar.

Didactic Courses and Course Development

The next major step in concept-based curriculum design is the development of courses that feature concepts and conceptual learning. Course learning outcomes are a starting point for course development. Unlike program learning outcomes that are not strikingly different in a concept-based curriculum compared with other curricular structures, course learning outcomes are different. They should clearly emphasize the application of concepts within the course and must link to the program learning outcomes. An example of a course learning outcome that might be developed within a concept-based curriculum (along with concepts and competencies) was presented earlier in this chapter (Table 4.1). Notice the linkages between course learning outcomes, competencies, concepts, and program learning outcomes. More detail regarding writing learning outcomes is presented in Chapter 7.

Many additional variables influence the direction of the curriculum when considering course design. First, the type of degree offered drives the total number of credit hours; thus the number of credits for nursing courses will vary. Also, the institution may influence some of the courses offered and the sequencing of those courses. The semester that students are admitted to the nursing program (e.g., direct entry, entry after the first semester, entry after 1 year, or entry after 2 years) must also be considered. Finally, the prerequisites and corequisites influence what is considered primary content or review content. For example, if anatomy, physiology, and pathophysiology are prerequisite courses taken before entry into the nursing curriculum, the courses designed for conceptual teaching will look different than if information from these courses were to be integrated into the nursing courses. After those things are considered, a decision must be made about how the concepts will be used within the courses. Two common paths may be taken: integrated into traditional population-focused and topic-focused courses, or as concept-focused courses.

Integration Into Population-Focused and Topic-Focused Courses. For years, nursing curricula have arranged content around population (such as pediatric, maternal child, adult, and geriatrics) and topic areas (such as mental health, leadership, and community). When this approach is used for a concept-based curriculum, concepts serve as a common link between and among courses. For example, all of the health and illness concepts apply to all population groups and thus are the core organizers of content for these courses. The focus for the concept presentation and exemplars are

TABLE 4.6 ■ **Sample of Course Arrangement in a Concept-Based Curriculum for a Four-Semester Nursing Program (upper division)**

SEMESTER 1	SEMESTER 2
Nursing Skills and Assessment Lab Patient Attributes Concepts Health and Illness Concepts I Clinical Practicum I	Health and Illness Concepts II Professional Nursing Concepts I Evidence-Based Nursing Practice Clinical Practicum II
SEMESTER 3	**SEMESTER 4**
Health and Illness Concepts III Professional Nursing Concepts II Clinical Practicum III Clinical Practicum IV	Global Health Concept Synthesis Clinical Practicum V Capstone

based on the population-specific elements for that concept. Professional nursing concepts fit into many of the fundamentals and leadership-type courses. In this approach, clinical courses continue to be closely linked to the traditional population-focused didactic courses.

One advantage to the population-focused and topic-focused approach is that many of the courses and clinical experiences maintain a level of familiarity and may be more readily accepted by faculty. A drawback to this approach is that faculty are tempted to change very little and claim they teach the concepts while continuing to overload students with content. Also, there is the potential for each faculty member in each course to teach the concept overview, which would result in duplication of effort.

MISCONCEPTIONS AND CLARIFICATIONS

Misconception: A simple way to develop a concept-based curriculum is to identify major concepts within courses of an existing curriculum.

Clarification: Designing a concept-based curriculum does not occur by simply identifying concepts in an existing curriculum, nor does it occur by adding concepts to an existing curriculum (i.e., an "add-on" approach). In concept-based curricula, concepts provide the structural framework for courses and content. Courses are redesigned with a specific plan for integration of concepts within the concepts.

Concept-Focused Courses. Another approach is to develop concept-focused courses that feature an integration of population groups. Courses may follow the identified concept categories (Table 4.6). For example, there may be a series of courses that feature health and illness concepts, a series of courses that feature professional nursing concepts, and a course that features health care recipient concepts. If macroconcepts are identified within concept categories, these may also be useful to consider so that concepts that are closely related are taught in a similar course.

When a concept-focused course approach is used, concepts and the dedicated exemplars are featured once in the designated didactic course. Thereafter the concepts are presented as interrelated concepts. Conceptual links across population groups and types of settings are made. Clinical courses should be designed to follow concept courses, and should apply concepts from *all* courses (health and illness, professional nursing concepts, and health care recipient concepts) into the clinical experience. In other words, clinical education represents the application and synthesis of all concepts, not just one group of concepts, in a variety of clinical sites and working with a variety of patient populations.

The benefit to this approach is that the concept is presented in greater depth, allowing for a deeper understanding to occur through exemplar reinforcement. However, this approach is not without challenges. It requires a very different teaching expectation among faculty and may result in the need for team teaching in the didactic courses. For example, the concept of *Gas Exchange* may be easy enough to teach, but the exemplars are likely to be representative of the health conditions across the age span, such as asthma in children and pneumonia in older adults. This approach also deemphasizes specialty content, and thus it is important that students have varied clinical experiences so they have clinical exposure across populations and specialties.

In addition to concept-featured courses, consideration of other types of courses should be included. As an example, a fundamentals course that teaches basic nursing skills and health assessment skills may still be necessary. In a baccalaureate curriculum, faculty may wish to offer a separate course focusing on community-based nursing, public health nursing, or nursing research. When this is the case, applicable core concepts are still to be woven into these courses.

Clinical Courses

Decisions about design of clinical courses are just as important as didactic course decisions. Furthermore, specific clinical learning activities (including simulation) should be incorporated into the overall curriculum plan. The conceptual approach offers an opportunity to break away from the traditional clinical education model that has been in place for well over 50 years. The emphasis has historically been placed on inpatient clinical courses that focus on caring for an assigned patient or patients, mimicking the work assignments of staff nurses in a designated clinical focus area. Students typically go to the unit to meet their assigned patient, review the medical record, and prepare required clinical paperwork prior to their clinical experience. During the clinical day, students receive, report, and care for their assigned patient(s), which may include the following activities: hygiene care, toileting, activity and exercise patient assessment, nutrition and dietary needs, medication administration, and a number of other interventions ordered by the physician. For many care activities, direct supervision by the nursing instructor or a primary nurse is required. Throughout the program, the advancement of clinical expertise is measured by the number and complexity of the patients assigned, and the gradual increase in competence and independence demonstrated by the student in the provision of care. Although direct patient care activities (DPCAs) such as the "patient of the day" approach still holds value, there are some clear downsides, including a tendency for students to focus on tasks and considerable downtime experienced by students as they wait for the necessary supervision (by an instructor or primary nurse) to complete nursing intervention (such as a dressing change or administering a medication). This type of clinical learning should be considered one teaching strategy among many other strategies used for clinical education.

Clinical courses designed for a concept-based curriculum include a variety of learning opportunities for students to apply several concepts in a number of ways and in a number of clinical situations. Clinical courses should link to didactic courses in that the application of concepts from the corequisite didactic courses should be emphasized. The learning activities can vary from the standard DPCA "patient of the day" to a multitude of "concept-focused" learning within the clinical area—also known as *focused clinical learning activities*. As an example, students might be assigned to study the concepts of *Immunity, Inflammation,* and *Infection* within a designated group of patients, and also consider how the concepts of *Health Policy* and *Health Care Economics* apply to the patient situations. Learning focuses on comparing and contrasting evidence of positive or ineffective immune status and evidence of, or risk for, inflammation and infection (among multiple patients) and includes the reinforcement of previously learned or new exemplars representing those concepts. Students might be asked to review policies that impact the care, as well as to compare health payment plans of the patients they are caring for. Simulation, with an emphasis on specified concepts, is another type of clinical learning activity that is effective. (Additional examples of concept-based teaching strategies for clinical education are presented in Chapter 7.)

Students should still have clinical experiences and exposure to various population groups and settings (e.g., pediatrics, adults, geriatrics, mental health, intensive care, and community) but with less emphasis placed on marching all students through the exact same set of clinical experiences. For example, in some programs offering a concept-based curriculum, students have an opportunity to choose the clinical courses (known as clinical intensives) that appeal to them after completing foundational clinical courses. Thus, in a given semester, students in the same cohort are applying concepts from the didactic concept courses in different clinical areas. Such an approach allows greater flexibility and efficiency in the way clinical sites are used (Giddens et al., 2008).

Tips for Success: Developing and Implementing the Concept-Based Curriculum

Most faculty are aware of the significant effort associated with developing and implementing a new curriculum. This section offers specific tips for enhancing success.

EXPECT A RANGE OF EMOTIONS

The reaction and emotions expressed among faculty will range from being thrilled about the change to being angry. Occasionally, opposing faculty may be disruptive to the work. Supporting faculty may become concerned if they are unable to gain full consensus among the faculty. Although this would be ideal, in most cases it is unrealistic. It is important that support for the curriculum work reaches *critical mass* to move forward, and energy should be directed toward working with those who seek change.

MANAGING RESISTANCE

Any new curriculum (especially a concept-based curriculum) represents significant effort from the curriculum committee and for faculty assigned to teach new courses. This can be threatening because nurse educators are forced to step out of their teaching comfort zone. Resistance to change is a natural reaction (particularly when the proposed change is not universally or well understood). Anticipating and accepting resistance as a normal part of the process is helpful so that strategies can be developed to ensure forward movement. Resistance is usually put forth by one or more strongly vested faculty who defend the old curriculum. Common arguments against change (presented below) can be easily countered by using non-adversarial responses.

"We Have Always Done It This Way! Why Should We Change?"

Extensive changes in health care, coupled with a growing call for change, makes this argument easy to address. Two early reports from the IOM, *Crossing the Quality Chasm* (IOM, 2001) and *Health Professions Education* (IOM, 2003), call for improvements to be made in health sciences education to improve quality of care. Specifically, several competencies such as patient-centered care, evidence-based medicine, working as part of an interdisciplinary team, focusing on quality improvement, and using information technology were emphasized, along with the need to address changing student demographics and teaching using active learning strategies (IOM, 2003). More recently, one of four key messages in the *Future of Nursing* report (IOM, 2010) is the need for nurses to achieve higher levels of education through *an improved education system* that promotes seamless academic progression. Another landmark publication, *Educating Nurses* (Benner, 2010), also describes the need for radical transformation of the education of nurses. A focus on and delivery of content in the traditional way does little to prepare nurses for the "situated cognition and action" needed for clinical practice (Benner, 2010, p. 13). Although these reports do not specify that a conceptual approach is needed, they all emphasize the need for an improved education system for effective health care delivery. In other words, the traditional approach to nursing education is outdated and is no longer preparing nurses adequately for the current health care system. It is simply the professional and ethical obligation of a higher-education professional to address and embrace this call for critical change within the nursing profession.

"Our NCLEX Pass Rates Are Good"

One of the biggest barriers to innovative curriculum work is the justifiable fear of reduced first-time pass rates on the National Council Licensure Examination (NCLEX). For years, first-time NCLEX pass rates have unofficially served as the gold standard measure of the quality of a nursing program. The Boards of Nursing in all states closely monitor first-time pass rates, setting a minimum standard expected of schools—which in some cases may create additional concern. In truth, the first-time NCLEX pass rate is only one indicator of program quality considered by accreditors. Other important measures include student and program measures. Examples of student measures include evidence of achievement of program outcomes, competencies, and student learning outcomes within courses, time to graduation, graduation rates, and the diversity of student enrollment. Program measures include an adequate number of qualified full-time faculty for the program(s) offered; tracking, orientation, and evaluation of preceptors and adjunct faculty; integrity of the curriculum; and a systematic approach to curriculum evaluation. The point is, a nursing program can have excellent first-time pass rates and yet can fail to address the changing needs of the nursing workforce. There is no intent to suggest that concept-based curricula will increase first-time pass rates, but no evidence exists that programs with a concept-based curriculum have a lower pass rate. In a survey of 57 nursing programs offering a concept-based curriculum, 35% reported higher first-time pass rates, 42% reported no changes in first-time pass rates, and 5% reported lower first-time pass rates. Eighteen percent of respondents did not know the impact on first-time pass rates (many had not yet graduated students from their new concept-based curriculum (Sportsman, 2013). Additionally, there have been five published studies in the nursing literature that have specifically reported NCLEX pass rates after implementing a concept-based curriculum. In four of the five studies, no significant change in NCLEX pass rates were reported (Duncan & Schultz, 2015; Lewis, 2014; Murray, Laurent, & Gontarz, 2015; and Patterson, Crager, Farmer, Epps, & Schuessler, 2016). One published study (Giddens & Morton, 2010) reported a drop in NCLEX pass rates with the first graduating cohort with a return to pre-curriculum change pass rates in subsequent cohorts.

"What Evidence Proves the Conceptual Approach Is Better?"

It is interesting that this question is raised over and over again, especially when there is plenty of evidence that our traditional approaches to educating the health care workforce have not been effective for the changing health care environment (Benner, 2010; IOM, 2001, 2003, 2010). One can defend the traditional approach by citing "evidence" based on first-time NCLEX pass rates, as though this is the only evidence that counts, but, as noted above, this argument does not hold. Although there is no "proof" that a conceptual approach for nursing education is better, the education discipline has plenty of evidence regarding improvements in learning and improvements in content management when the conceptual approach is applied (Ambrose et al., 2010; Erikson, 2002; Erikson, 2008; Schmidt, McKnight, & Raizen, 1997; Sousa, 2010; Zull, 2002). Over time, as more nurse educators adopt the conceptual approach, we can expect the availability of published program and student learning outcomes.

"Our Faculty Workloads Are Too Heavy"

The nationwide faculty shortage has several implications for nursing programs, but what is especially problematic is the effect on faculty work assignments. It is unlikely that any nursing program has faculty who are not concerned about the amount of work associated with their jobs. Thus, this is a statement and argument that is universally heard with any project, initiative, or change introduced to faculty groups. It is true that adopting the conceptual approach initially requires significant effort—not only with curriculum development, but also to change teaching. However, over time faculty learn how to effectively teach conceptually, and often they find that the teaching effort is more effective and efficient.

An expectation of all faculty, regardless of the type of institution or type of discipline, is maintaining currency in educational delivery. Curriculum development and advancing one's teaching should not be presented as an "add-on" or "additional work"—rather, this should be presented as a professional obligation to the students, institution, and profession. Furthermore, once the curriculum is developed and faculty begin the process of transitioning their teaching practice, there is often a level of energy and excitement that is associated with the teaching-learning process.

SECURE RESOURCES

Undertaking any major effort is met with greater acceptance if adequate resources are available. Examples of helpful resources include:

- Expert consultation from nursing faculty experienced in the development of a concept-based curriculum or consultation from faculty in other disciplines, such as education
- Site visits to nursing programs that have successfully adopted a concept-based curriculum
- A dedicated work assignment for key faculty who are leading the curriculum change
- Faculty development opportunities, especially in the area of concept-based teaching and learning
- Support from senior administrators in the nursing program, particularly for additional help needed or flexibility in teaching assignments, admissions, and course scheduling as the new curriculum is rolled out

EXPECT HARD WORK AND ENCOURAGE AND SUPPORT ONE ANOTHER

Curriculum redesign is very challenging work that takes a great deal of time. Faculty should not begin with an expectation that the process will be completed quickly. A great deal of discussion, negotiating, and reflection is needed at the beginning of the process to elicit input and build the initial support needed to begin work, let alone the numerous meetings and work needed for the actual curriculum design. Developing a trusting, encouraging, and supportive relationship among the faculty—particularly those directly involved in the curriculum work—helps to sustain the effort needed over time.

ENGAGE YOUR CLINICAL PARTNERS

Collaborating with nurses in practice settings (particularly those from clinical agencies where students complete clinical experiences) in the development and implementation of the curriculum can enrich the work and deepen the relationships between the nursing school and the clinical agency. Eliciting input and support from these important stakeholders during the process increases the level of acceptance of the planned changes. This is particularly important when redesigning clinical education and attempting to implement significantly different learning activities within the various clinical sites.

Summary

This chapter has reviewed the general steps associated with the development of a concept-based curriculum. Some of the most important points to reiterate about this process include:

1. The general curriculum development process is the same—it is the curriculum design that is unique.
2. Concepts used for the curriculum represent concepts of nursing practice as opposed to concepts representing the discipline of nursing from a theoretical perspective.
3. Content saturation is avoided by carefully considering the concepts and the number of exemplars to include in the curriculum.
4. Course design (including clinical course design) and teaching practices will change.
5. The process is difficult and often is met with resistance. Resistance is not a reason to abandon the idea but rather represents a difference in the values and perspectives of faculty. The lack of understanding related to the conceptual approach is often the greatest source of resistance.

References

Ambrose SA, Bridges MW, DiPietro M, Lovett MC, Norman MK. *How Learning Works. 7 Research-Based Principles for Smart Teaching.* San Francisco, CA: John Wiley & Sons; 2010.

Bastable S. *Nurse as Educator.* 4th ed. Sudbury, MA: Jones & Bartlett; 2013.

Benner P, Sutphen M, Leonard V, Day L. *Educating Nurses: A Call for Radical Transformation.* San Francisco, CA: Josey-Bass; 2010.

Boland DL. Developing curriculum: frameworks, outcomes and competencies. In: Billings D, Halstead J, eds. *Teaching in Nursing.* 4th ed. St. Louis, MO: Elsevier; 2012.

Boland DL. Program Evaluation and public accountability. In: Oermann M, Heinrich K, eds. *Annual Review of Nursing Education.* New York, NY: Springer; 2004.

Caputi L. Curriculum design and development. In: Caputi L, ed. *Teaching Nursing: The Art and Science.* Vol. 1. 2nd ed. Chicago, IL: College of DuPage; 2010.

Csokasy J. A congruent curriculum: philosophical integrity from philosophy to outcomes. *J Nurs Educ.* 2002;41:469–470.

Duncan K, Schulz PS. Impact of change to a concept-based baccalaureate nursing curriculum on student and program outcomes. *J Nurs Educ.* 2015;54(3):S16–S20.

Erikson L. *Concept-Based Curriculum and Instruction.* Thousand Oaks, CA: Corwin Press; 2002.

Erikson L. *Stirring the Head, Heart, and Soul: Redefining Curriculum, Instruction, and Concept-Based Learning.* Thousand Oaks, CA: Corwin Press; 2008.

Giddens J, Brady D, Brown P, Wright M, Smith D, Harris J. A new curriculum for a new era of nursing education. *Nurs Educ Perspect.* 2008;29:200–204.

Giddens J, Morton N. Report card: an evaluation of a concept-based curriculum. *Nurs Educ Perspect.* 2010;31:372–377.

Giddens J, Wright M, Gray I. Selecting concepts for a concept-based curriculum: application of a benchmark approach. *J Nurs Educ.* 2012;51:511–515.

Goudreau J, Pepin J, Dubois S, Boyer L, Larue C, Legault A. A second generation of the competency-based approach to nursing education. *Int J Nurs Educ Scholarsh.* 2009;6(1).

Institute of Medicine. *Crossing the Quality Chasm.* Washington, DC: National Academies Press; 2001.

Institute of Medicine. *Health Professions Education.* Washington, DC: National Academies Press; 2003.

Institute of Medicine. *The Future of Nursing: Leading Change, Advancing Health.* Washington, DC: National Academies Press; 2010.

Interprofessional Education Collaboration Expert Panel. *Core Competencies for Interprofessional Collaborative Practice: Report of an Expert Panel.* Washington DC: Interprofessional Education Collaborative; 2011.

Lewis L. Outcomes of a concept-based curriculum. *Teach Learn Nurs.* 2014;9:75–79.

Murray S, Laurent K, Gontarz J. Evaluation of a concept-based curriculum: a tool and process. *Teach Learn Nurs.* 2015;10:169–175.

Nelson ML, Howell JK, Larson JC, Karpiuk KL. Student outcomes of the healing web: evaluation of a transformative model for nursing education. *J Nurs Educ*. 2001;40:404–413.

Patterson LD, Crager JM, Farmer A, Epps CD, Schuessler JB. A strategy to ensure faculty engagement when assessing a concept-based curriculum. *J Nurs Educ*. 2016;55:467–470.

Quality and Safety Education in Nursing [QSEN] competencies, QSEN, n.d: Retrieved from: qsen.org/

Schmidt WH, McKnight CC, Raizen S. *A Splintered Vision: An Investigation of U.S. Science and Mathematics Education, U.S. National Research Center for the Third International Mathematics and Science Study (TIMSS)*. Dordrecht, Netherlands: Kluwer Academic Publishers; 1997.

Sousa DA. *Mind, Brain, and Education. Neuroscience Implications for the Classroom*. Bloomington, IL: Solution Tree Press; 2010.

Sportsman S, for the Academic Consulting Group. *Nationwide Concept Based Curriculum Survey Analysis* [PowerPoint presentation]. Amsterdam: Elsevier; 2013.

Sullivan DT. An introduction to curriculum development. In: Billings D, Halstead J, eds. *Teaching in Nursing*. 5th ed. St. Louis, MO: Elsevier; 2016.

Whittmann-Price RA, Fasolka BJ. Objectives and outcomes: the fundamental difference. *Nurs Educ Perspect*. 2010;31:233–236.

Zull JE. *The Art of the Changing Brain*. Sterling, VA: Stylus Publishing; 2002.

CHAPTER 5

Conceptual Learning

Jean Giddens

A key challenge shared among all instructors—regardless of the discipline or student level—is creating an optimal platform for learning. In higher education, faculty are primarily hired because of their expertise in their respective discipline and often lack an understanding of how people learn. Faculty tend to focus on honing a teaching style that works well for them, with little thought on how student learning occurs as a result of their efforts. A common assumption held by new and many seasoned instructors is that students learn as a result of attending a class or completing a course. The flaw in this thinking is nested in a general lack of understanding about what learning is and the science behind learning. The truth is, learning is not something that is "done" to students by instructors; rather, learning is something that students accomplish themselves. Instructors have a role in facilitating this process by creating purposeful and engaging learning activities in an optimal learning environment.

Conceptual learning was identified in Chapter 1 as one of five separate but interrelated elements associated with the conceptual approach. The desired outcome associated with conceptual learning is that students gain a deep understanding of concepts and the ability to transfer ideas to other situations through cognitive connections. Nurse educators adopting the conceptual approach are usually eager to learn how to teach conceptually. However, gaining an understanding of the science of learning is foundational to teaching. Put another way, the science of instruction builds on the science of learning. Having an understanding about how learning occurs must precede conversations about best teaching practices. In this chapter, principles associated with the science of learning will be presented, along with the linkages to the conceptual approach.

Definition of Learning and Learning Theories

There are many definitions of learning representing a wide range of perspectives. Ambrose and colleagues offer a contemporary definition reflective of the science of learning. They define learning as "a *process* that leads to *change* which occurs as a result of *experience* and increases the potential for improved performance and future learning" (Ambrose, Bridges, Dipietro, Lovett, & Norman, 2010, p. 3). Emphasis on the words "process," "change," and "experience" represents three key components of the definition. *Process* is emphasized because learning is a brain-based physiological process that occurs in the mind. Learning cannot be directly seen or measured, but inferences that learning has occurred are made based on student performance. *Change* is emphasized because learning results in a change in students' knowledge, beliefs, behaviors, attitudes, and values. Although the change occurs over time, an enduring impact occurs. *Experience* is emphasized because learning is shaped by the interpretation and response to former and current experiences. Experiences take on many forms, some more powerful than others. In any given situation, students may or may not be aware of the influence of experiences on their learning. These key components become clearer in the sections that follow. How learning actually occurs has been debated for years, and, as a result, multiple classic

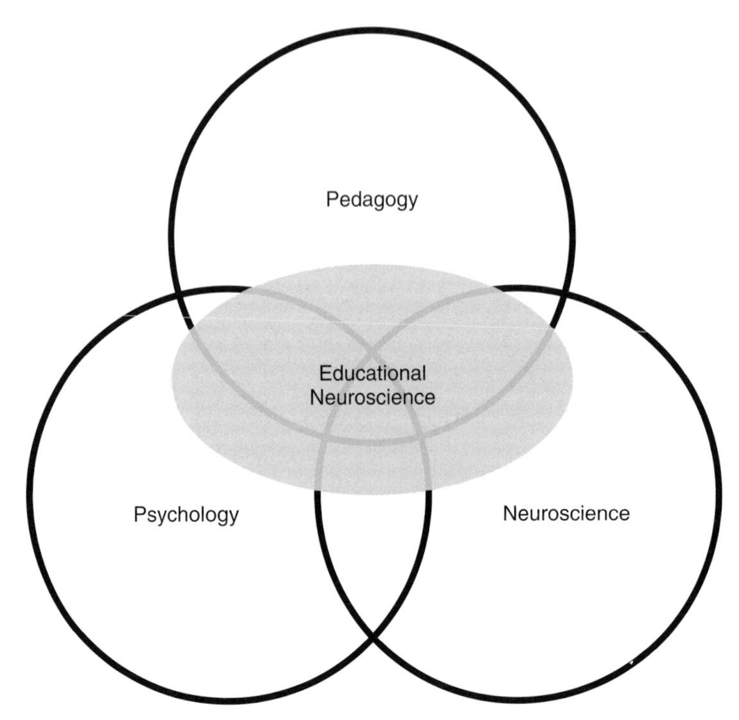

Fig. 5.1 Educational neuroscience represents pedagogy, neuroscience, and psychology.

learning theories have been proposed, including behaviorist, cognitivism, constructivism, cognitive development, and humanism. During the past few decades, there has been increasing interest in neuroscience and brain-based learning theories, grounded in the premise that biologic changes in the brain occur in response to learning. The intent of this chapter is not to present all learning theories but rather to use neuroscience and brain-based theory to explain conceptual learning.

Educational Neuroscience: How the Brain Learns

Although the majority of brain development occurs as part of prenatal development through early childhood, the brain continues to develop, adapt, and change in response to learning throughout life. Learning is a complex process with multiple variables. *Educational neuroscience* is a term used to describe the interrelationship between neuroscience, teaching practices, and psychology as key components of the learning process (Figure 5.1). Essentially, the premise of educational neuroscience is that learning involves physiological changes within the brain (primarily through changes in neural circuitry) and that the learning environment, instruction methods, and psychological factors of the learner influence the learning process. A significant focus of educational neuroscience is on the optimal conditions for the brain to learn (Ambrose, Bridges, Dipietro, Lovett, & Normal, 2010; Connell, 2009; Jensen, 2008; Sosa, 2010). Learning is optimal when the brain is in a calm, relaxed state, where the active learning is challenging (but not threatening), when multiple experiences are provided in a realistic context, and when the learner is required to connect to previous knowledge.

It is imperative that all educators gain an understanding of these components to fully grasp how to effectively facilitate conceptual learning. In the sections that follow, a very brief review of brain structures and function is included as a foundation for understanding the process of learning. The discussion of brain function is only done with the intent to explain how the brain learns.

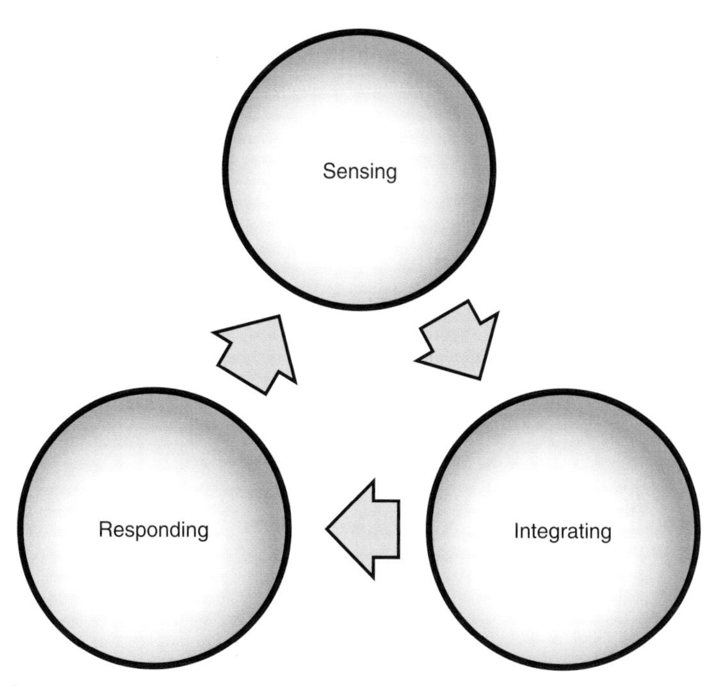

Fig. 5.2 Sensing, integrating, and responding are ongoing and continuous processes within the brain.

GENERAL BRAIN FUNCTION

A very simplistic summarization of what the brain does can be described in three words: *sensing*, *integrating*, and *responding*. **Sensing** refers to an ongoing process whereby the brain takes in data signals (input) from a variety of internal (physiological) and external (environmental) sources. The brain interfaces with millions of data signals, most of which do not require conscious thought. **Integrating** is the process of sorting and grouping data and then making sense of those data. This data sorting occurs immediately and does not require purposeful thought. Put another way, integration is the process of brain recognition and interpretation that occurs with the sum of all the data signals (Zull, 2002). **Responding** refers to the outcome of the data integration. Based on the sorting and grouping of data signals, the brain sends information to target areas, triggering a wide variety of physiological responses, including regulatory and motor responses (voluntary and automatic movements). The transfer of data signals—from sensory input, integration, to response—is continuous, cyclic, and automatic; sensory input triggers integrative activity, which triggers physiological and motor response (Figure 5.2).

Brain Structures

The brain is a highly complex structure within the central nervous system and is composed of three major units: the cerebrum, the brainstem, and the cerebellum. The cerebrum comprises the largest part of the human brain and is divided into two hemispheres (right and left), each of which are divided into four lobes (frontal, temporal, parietal, and occipital) as shown in Figure 5.3. The outer layer covering the cerebrum is the cortex; together, these are referred to as the *cerebral cortex*. Neurons within the cortex are responsible for many of the highly sophisticated aspects of cognitive functioning. The limbic system is a group of structures that connect higher and lower brain functions (Figure 5.4). Together these structures regulate emotion, mood, pleasure, and motivation.

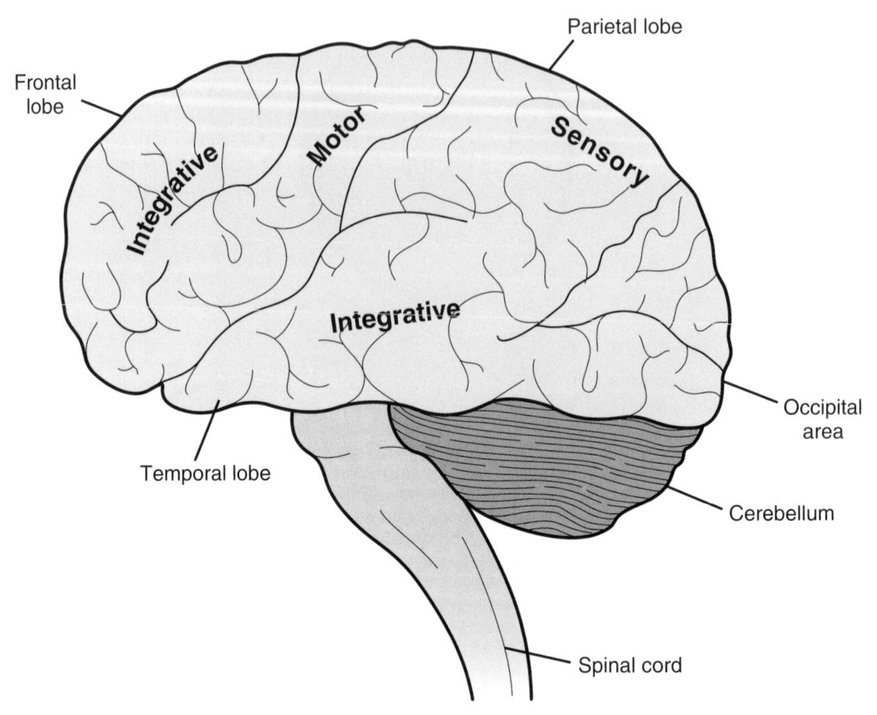

Fig. 5.3 Structures of the outer brain and functional areas for sensory, integrative, and motor functions.

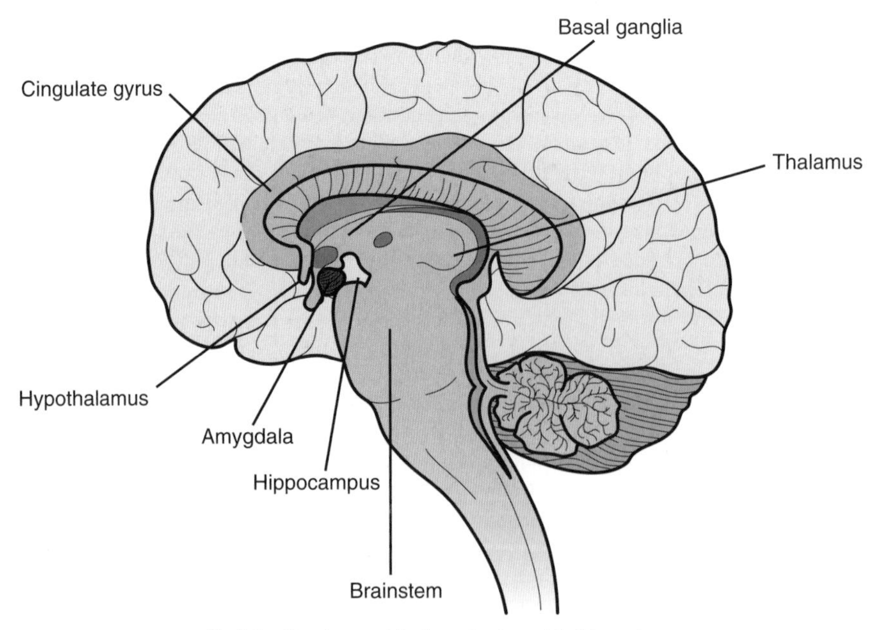

Fig. 5.4 Structures of the inner brain and limbic system.

BOX 5.1 ■ Limbic Structure Functions

- The *basal ganglia* are paired structures that are involved with automatic and voluntary movement.
- The *thalamus* is a relay center and transfers nearly all signals to the cerebral cortex.
- The *hypothalamus* regulates the autonomic nervous system and the endocrine system.
- The *amygdala* is a walnut-sized structure that influences emotional states on sensory input and has a role in determining what memories retained. This structure has tremendous influence on learning.
- The *hippocampus* plays a significant role in information transfer to long-term memory.
- The *cingulate gyrus* serves as a message transfer channel to and from the limbic system.

Box 5.1 presents a review of limbic structure functions. The brainstem, located at the base of the brain, includes the midbrain, pons, and medulla. The cerebellum, tucked behind the brainstem and beneath the occipital lobe of the cerebrum, coordinates movement and equilibrium (see Figure 5.3).

Neurons

At the cellular level, neurons are built for efficiency in transmitting information. Neurons have three functional characteristics: (1) generate nerve impulses, (2) transmit nerve impulse to other parts of the cell, and (3) transmit signals to other cells and organs to create an effect. Neurons direct signals from cell to cell through dendrites and axons. Axons of one cell extend to the dendrites of the next cell (Figure 5.5). Signals are sent back and forth from cell to cell across the synapse, the gap between axons and dendrites. The process is enhanced by the myelin sheath—a coating over the axon and neurotransmitters. It is estimated that the human brain has more than 100 billion neurons, with as many as 10,000 connections per neuron! Connections become a very important point in the next section when considering the brain structures related to learning.

BRAIN STRUCTURES AND LEARNING

Obviously, the brain is far more complex in its function and structure than the preceding discussion would suggest. However, this simplified approach (sensing, integrating, and responding) provides a useful framework for understanding the science of learning because the same process supports learning. The primary activity of human learning involves taking data in, integrating the data for meaning, and responding. These functions occur through trillions of data signals and networks between the neurons within the cerebral cortex. Various areas of the cerebral cortex play specific roles in the process of sensing, integrating, and responding as it relates to learning.

The function of sensing involves receiving auditory, visual, olfactory, and tactile data signals. The thalamus, located at the base of the cerebrum (see Fig. 5.4), serves as the brain's primary dispatch center for sensory data. It sends data signals (which are essentially nothing more than isolated bits of data) to the temporal and frontal regions of the cerebral cortex for integration.

The integrative process involves merging these data into clusters that become meaningful, such as visual recognition, language, sound, and images. These meanings are further integrated in various ways that become thoughts, ideas, and plans for action (Zull, 2002). Considering the physiological function of various areas of the cerebrum, this process makes a great deal of sense. The frontal lobe is responsible for memory retention, higher level cognitive function, expressive speech, and voluntary eye and motor movement, while the temporal lobe controls receptive speech and the integration of visual, somatic and auditory data. Interpretation of spatial data information occurs within the sensory cortex of the parietal lobe, while the processing of visual data occurs in the occipital lobe.

Responding refers to carrying out the action plans formed in the integration phase. Located centrally within the cerebrum are the paired basal ganglia, which are responsible for the initiation, execution,

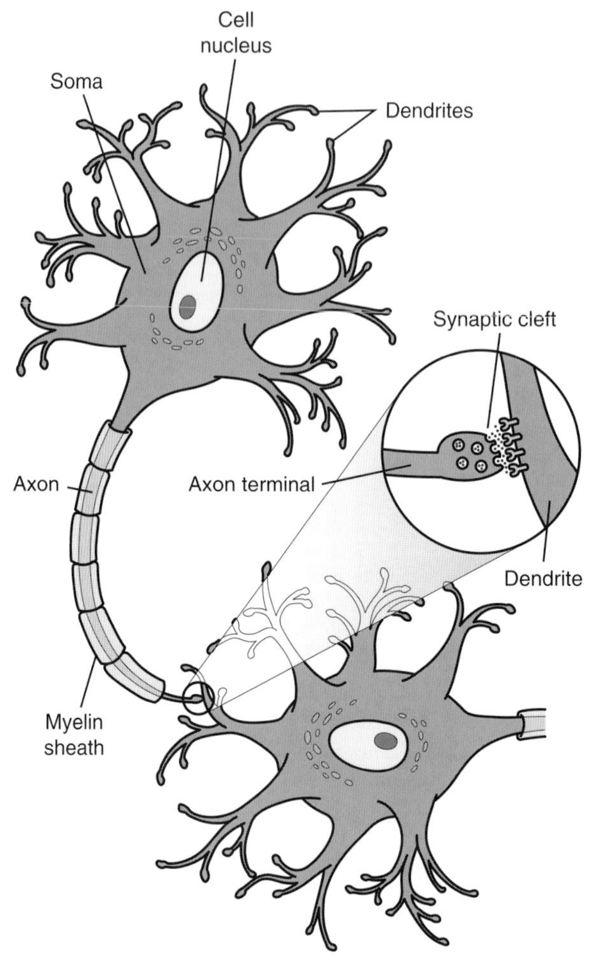

Fig. 5.5 Structure of a neuron. (From Heuston, DH, with JW Parkinson. *The Third Source: A Message of Hope for Education.* UT: Author; 2011: p. 235.)

and completion of voluntary and automatic movement. These movements are necessary for a variety of actions, from blinking, swallowing, running, scratching, and—more specifically related to learning—the formation of speech and the ability to write, draw, and perform other related movements. The transfer of data signals (sensory input, integration, and motor response) is continuous and cyclic; sensory input triggers integrative activity, which triggers motor activity. The motor activity in turn serves as sensory data that start the cycle again. This cycle is automatic, and to a large extent it is subconscious. Figure 5.6 shows the pattern and flow of sensory input, data integration, and motor response across the brain.

THE LEARNING BRAIN

Sensing, Integrating, and Responding

Learning involves a combination of taking in new information and active thinking to translate that information into meaning and appropriate actions. The three elements of sensing, integrating, and responding once again apply to this discussion.

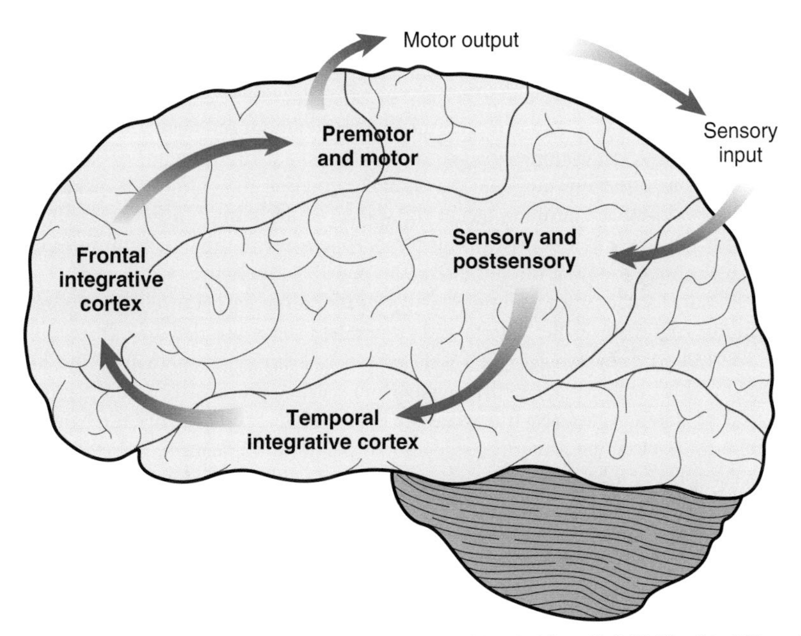

Fig. 5.6 Sensory input, data integration, and motor response. (Modified from Zull JE. *The Art of Changing the Brain: Enriching the Practice of Teaching by Exploring the Biology of Learning*. Sterling, VA: Stylus Publishing, LLC; 2002.)

In a learning situation, new information presents as auditory, visual, olfactory, and tactile data signals. The intake of information from the sensing brain has limited benefit or use unless the information is applied. In other words, there must be a process whereby the student not only receives knowledge but also uses the knowledge in a way that requires the brain to actively integrate the information so it can be transformed into understanding and meaning. Little is gained in situations where there is an intake of new information without using that information to stimulate thinking, create ideas, or generate an action plan.

Based on the preceding discussion, it should be obvious that integration of information is a necessary step for learning to take place. Referring back to the previous section, two areas of the brain are involved with integration. The temporal integrative cortex involves memory of places and stories and information as facts. When new information comes in, the learner builds on existing knowledge—through existing neuronal networks. The frontal integrative cortex involves active mental energy, decisions, choice, and creativity. For this reason, learning is enhanced when there is balance between the two integrative sections. The outcome of a balanced approach is the transformation of a learner from a receiver of information to a producer of ideas (Zull, 2002).

Extending Neural Connections

The term *neuroplasticity* is used to describe the brain's ability to reorganize and restructure itself through the formation of new neural connections as a result of experiences (Dragansk & Gaser, 2004). Neuroplasticity is an outcome of effective learning. When the brain is challenged with new information and problem solving, the integrative process of the mind involves clustering of data. In other words, the brain looks for patterns for meaningful organization and categorization of the information. New knowledge and information is matched to memory, extending neural networks. This process facilitates the construction and extension of neuron connections; new knowledge structures are built with a new baseline for incoming information.

Seeking patterns represents an important underlying process associated with brain efficiency. The brain seeks patterns based on previous learning and experiences, allowing for very efficient responses to acquired knowledge and efficiency in extending knowledge with new information. However, sometimes mistakes are made with initial interpretation, and further information may be needed for clarification. For example, if a person walking on a path through the woods encounters an object that is long and thin, the brain may initially interpret the object as a snake resulting in a fear response, and perhaps jumping out of the way to avoid harm. On further evaluation, it is determined that the shape is just a stick. This response results from the brain misinterpreting the visual cue and forming an initial response based on previous experiences with snakes. Likewise, a person may initially misidentify a wild raspberry plant for poison ivy because the brain searches for patterns—in this case three-leaflet pattern and growth in a shady wooded area. It requires further inspection and additional knowledge (such as the presence of thorny stems) to make the distinction.

Similarly, mistakes can be made in the thinking and learning process when information is incorrectly interpreted; this is particularly true when the brain anticipates something else based on preestablished patterns. For example, a nursing student may fail to notice nuances in drug administration information, particularly if he or she lacks awareness of such differences. Thus the brain may incorrectly interpret new information based on preformed patterns. This is especially problematic if the student has built patterns on inaccurate or incomplete information. As an example, a student may believe that poor health outcomes among underrepresented minorities is based on genetic differences or their failure to take advantage of health services available to them. This information base must be clarified in order for the student to develop an accurate conceptual understanding of health disparities.

Variables Influencing Learning

EMOTION

Earlier in this chapter, education neuroscience was introduced and described as an interrelationship between neuroscience, teaching, and psychological influences of the learner. Emotion represents a key psychological influence on the learner. It has been noted several times throughout this chapter that sensing is one of the primary functions of the brain, and this involves the input of information. The emotional state of the learner influences the way sensory data are filtered in the brain. A positive emotional state favors conduction through the amygdala, and, as a result, information reaches the integrative areas of the brain. Positive states also enhance memory retention, particularly when there is something novel about the learning activity. These effects have been shown through neuroimaging studies (Pawlak, Margarinos, Melchor, McEwen, & Strickland, 2003). In times of stress, fear, or anger, sensory data are largely sent to the lower-level reactive brain and data are not available for higher cognitive processing (Willis, 2010). This mechanism explains why it is very difficult to focus and learn in times of extreme stress and why individuals are more likely to be productive and learn when they are in a positive emotional state. The amygdala also has a powerful effect in committing emotionally charged events (both positive and negative) to long-term memory. This phenomenon can be better understood by recalling a very happy, sad, or scary event in your life. Details of such events are often easy to recall, even decades later.

Strategies to support the emotional regulation of learners has been described by L. Kuypers (2011) in her framework outlined in the curriculum, The Zones of Regulation (www.zonesofregulation.com). The four zones range from Blue, Green, Yellow, and Red Zone Table 5.1. The Green Zone represents a state where the learner has an optimal level of alertness for academic pursuits, is relaxed, focused, and open to learning. Peak learning occurs in the Green Zone because a positive and calm emotional state allows information to reach the integrative areas of the brain, optimizing

TABLE 5.1 ■ **Zones of Regulation and Learning**

Zone	Alertness and Emotional State	Effect on Learning
Blue Zone	Low state of alertness; sadness, boredom, sleepy.	Suboptimal learning
Green Zone	Calm, relaxed state.	Optimal learning
Yellow Zone	Heightened state of alertness; anxiety, stress, excessive happiness.	Suboptimal learning
Red Zone	Extreme state; anger, rage, terror, devastation.	Learning not possible

The Zones of Regulation® and Learning.

thinking and memory retention. The Blue Zone represents a low state of alertness and is associated with feelings of sadness, depression, not feeling well, fatigue, sleepiness, or boredom. Learners in a Blue Zone are exposed to information, but because they are in a low state of alertness, the data signals may not effectively reach a high-level integration state. Learners may also struggle to recall information. Individuals in a Blue state need to "recharge" and this partly explains the need for engaging educational approaches, and the need for periodic breaks during learning. Alternatively, the Yellow Zone represents a heightened state of alertness and emotions, commonly associated with feelings of anxiety, stress, nervousness, frustration as well as excitement. Although learning may occur when a person is in the Yellow Zone, it often is not optimal academic performance. The Red Zone represents an extreme heightened state of alertness and extreme emotions such as terror, anger, rage, elation or devastation. It is rare that learning would occur when a person is in a Red Zone because data signals essentially are directed to the lower reactive brain as opposed to the integrative cortex for higher-level thinking.

DOPAMINE

Another key variable associated with learning is dopamine, a neurotransmitter that facilitates the transmission of signals between neurons in the brain. Dopamine produces pleasurable feelings and the amount of dopamine released is influenced by emotional states. An increased release of dopamine is triggered with positive experiences and a drop in dopamine release can occur with negative experiences (Willis, 2010). This is an important principle because of dopamine's influence on learning. Dopamine acts as a reward mechanism in the brain related to learning and enhances the brain's translation of the information to memory. The nucleus accumbens, a dopamine storage structure, has been shown to release more dopamine when learners get answers right (which in turn creates a pleasurable feeling). Likewise, less dopamine is released when learners make a mistake or get an answer wrong (Salamone & Correa, 2002). This reward occurs when the brain is challenged and successful when thinking about new information and solving new problems. Individuals with mastery in basic math would not get rewarded with increased dopamine release for correctly solving simple mathematical questions (such as $3 \times 5 = x$, or $12 + 6 = x$) because arriving at these answers does not represent a challenge. An individual is also not rewarded with dopamine when he or she attempts to solve a challenging problem and gets the answer wrong or is unable to make substantive progress. When there is no reward, motivation is reduced. Gee (2007) describes the power of this effect in the context of computer games with multiple levels that are increasingly challenging. The dopamine-enhanced pleasure of successfully achieving a level motivates the player to go on to the next, more challenging level.

MISCONCEPTIONS AND CLARIFICATIONS

Misconception: Rote memorization has no benefit to students and should be discouraged.

Clarification: Rote memorization of factual knowledge actually provides some benefits because base information is easily and efficiently retrieved by the brain. Gaining a deep understanding of concepts and the ability to make generalizations from this understanding is supported by accurate, factual information. Rote memorization of facts does not, in itself, lead to higher order thinking, but provides the foundation to do so. The goal is for *learning with understanding* as opposed to *remembering and repeating facts*.

MOVEMENT

Another variable that impacts learning is movement. It has been known for years that the brain is more active when the body is active and less active when the body is stationary (Sosa, 2010). Body movement increases the flow of blood to the brain, thereby increasing the delivery of oxygen and glucose to neurons. Movement also enhances the brain's access to long-term memory. Studies also have shown that increased brain mass, cognitive processing, and mood regulation are associated with exercise.

NUTRITION

The link between proper nutrition and peak learning has been well documented. Optimal neurotransmission within the brain requires adequate hydration. A reduced hydrated state can lead to poor concentration, emotional changes, and reduced cognitive abilities, all of which have a negative impact on the ability to learn. Carbohydrates are the main source of fuel for the brain. The importance of healthy carbohydrate choices is based on the evidence that wide fluctuations in sugar levels hamper effective neurotransmission. An intake of an excessive amount of simple sugar triggers insulin release, which can cause drowsiness. In contrast, complex carbohydrates are associated with a slower breakdown and absorption of sugar, providing a steady release of fuel. Fats and proteins are needed to enhance healthy neurons, which in turn impacts neurotransmission.

SLEEP

The sleep-deprived brain negatively impacts learning because of a lack of focus and attention. In this state, the brain has a reduced ability to take in (sense) data from learning situations. Furthermore, when a person is in a sleep-deprived state, neurons are unable to efficiently coordinate data impulses leading to impaired cognitive capacity. Sleep deprivation also impacts the brain's ability to store information into memory and memory recall. Committing something that has recently been learned to memory requires sleep—or, put another way, sleeping well the night after learning new information or a new skill is important for memory and future performance (Sosa, 2010). Memory consolidation (i.e., stabilization of a memory) takes place during sleep through the strengthening of neural connections. Although this process is poorly understood, it is thought that this process is linked to sleep waves during different phases of the sleep cycle. Memory recall (ie, the ability to access something previously stored into memory) is also negatively impacted with insufficient sleep. Several other negative impacts of sleep deprivation are reported in the literature, including mood. Specific to learning, sleep-deprived students tend to have lower grades and are more likely to be depressed compared with their peers who get adequate sleep (Wolfson & Carskadon, 1998).

Conceptual Learning in the Nursing Discipline

Throughout this chapter, the discussion has focused on the science of learning without specific reference to conceptual learning. The science of learning provides substantial evidence related to the benefits of conceptual learning. It should be increasingly clear that the conceptual approach is an opportunity for nurse educators to adopt strategies that enhance student learning. Ideally, this approach benefits learners not only while they are enrolled in nursing programs but also gives them the skills to emerge as efficient life-long learners throughout their career.

The massive volume of new knowledge generated throughout our society has made it impossible for any education program in any discipline to "cover" all the information in an academic program. With a greater understanding of how the brain learns, nursing educators must emphasize *learning with understanding* as opposed to *remembering and repeating facts*. Adopting the conceptual approach transforms the nursing education environment from a passive, static state with limited emotion or engagement into a vibrant, active, and challenging state with enhanced learning as an outcome. Given the preceding discussion about learning science, the relevance of this approach should be clear.

Timpson and Bendel-Simso (1996) described conceptual learning as a process by which students learn to organize information into logical mental structures and become increasingly skilled at thinking. Conceptual learning requires the application of concepts and conceptual understanding to a situation, but supported by a foundation of factual information. Thus a hallmark of conceptual learning is that it necessitates the use of facts as opposed to a focus on facts, and the use of facts should be within the application of information in a larger context. Put another way, a deep understanding of concepts and the ability to make generalizations from those concepts is supported by facts and factual learning (Erikson & Lanning, 2014). It is the interaction of facts and concepts, within the context of clinical situations that leads to deep understanding and the ability to transfer that information to other situations. Conceptual learning facilitates the formation of knowledge structures through neural connections and establishes patterns and connections in the brain. Over time, the conceptual learner develops an increased ability to translate previously learned information across multiple situations and context and also the ability to take in new information and make connections between similar ideas and situations. In nursing, learning experiences should ideally be placed in the context of a clinical situation and be purposeful—in other words, learners should clearly recognize the benefit of what they are learning and how it applies to the practice of nursing. Students must be exposed to clinical problems, and effective conceptual learning requires an investigative approach whereby they are challenged to think through multiple variables and to make important associations.

CONCEPTUAL THINKING AND EXPERT THINKING

As noted previously, the brain builds a network of new neural connections during the learning process. The conceptual approach cultivates this process because the learner is making connections by actively thinking about the interrelationships of information to concepts and the interface of concepts across multiple situations and contexts. Patricia Benner's classic work *From Novice to Expert* (Benner, 1984) presented narratives describing thinking approaches among nurses across a spectrum of five stages of expertise: novice, advanced beginner, competent, proficient, and expert. Expert nurses, using their enormous background of experiences, have an accurate and intuitive grasp of situations and know how to respond, even in unique situations not previously encountered. This ability comes from well-honed cognitive skills—that is, the ability to focus on important data and recognize situations, synthesizing and analyzing the meaning of those data, and connecting this information to previous knowledge and experiences for an appropriate and seamless response. Bransford, Brown, and Cocking (2000) point out that only a subset of one's total knowledge applies to any particular problem. Experts possess a rich and large reservoir of knowledge connected and organized around important concepts. They also have the skill to retrieve the applicable and appropriate knowledge related to a presenting problem, which is referred to as *conditionalized knowledge*. A key element of conceptual learning is honing the skill of conditionalized knowledge retrieval for problem solving.

Novices, by comparison, tend to have knowledge arranged in a list-like, disconnected fashion. They are unable to effortlessly and accurately respond to complex problems because they lack contextual experience, are more likely to have rigid or rule-based understanding of information, and tend to approach problem solving from a linear-thinking approach. New graduates who lack conceptual thinking skills are challenged during the transition to practice because they lack not only depth in clinical experiences but also the cognitive skills needed to make conceptual connections.

CONCEPTUAL LEARNING AND MEANINGFUL PATTERNS

A discussion regarding seeking patterns as a process associated with brain efficiency was presented earlier in this chapter. Conceptual organization allows an expert to see patterns and relationships not apparent to novice learners. Conceptual learning fosters the development of cognitive organization that is ultimately useful in specific contexts in which information is applicable, and it supports deep understanding. The organization of information into a conceptual framework allows for an enhanced ability to transfer and apply information to a new situation (Figure 5.7). The ability of the brain to transfer and apply information is hampered when knowledge lacks organization and presents as a set of disconnected facts. For this reason, a conceptual organization of information is foundational to clinical reasoning. The formation of clinical judgment and clinical reasoning in nursing requires an ability to make cognitive connections to past experiences and learn from new experiences, thus building the neural connections related to nursing expertise. Clinical judgement represents a desired outcome of conceptual learning because of the trajectory from learning facts, to thinking about concepts, and the ability to make generalizations and linkages to principles. Tanner's Model of Clinical Judgment (Tanner, 2006) presents this process as occurring from the perspective of noticing, interpreting, responding, and reflecting and doing so within situational context. The recognition of patterns related to specific conditions and situations is central to noticing and interpreting. This also closely links to the previous sections describing data intake and integrative processes within the brain. Responding represents the decision making and response that occurs in the brain. Reflecting, especially within the context of learning, represents the process of neuroplasticity (ie, the formation of new neural connections within the brain as a result of experiences). Reflecting on these experiences drives deeper understanding for future learning.

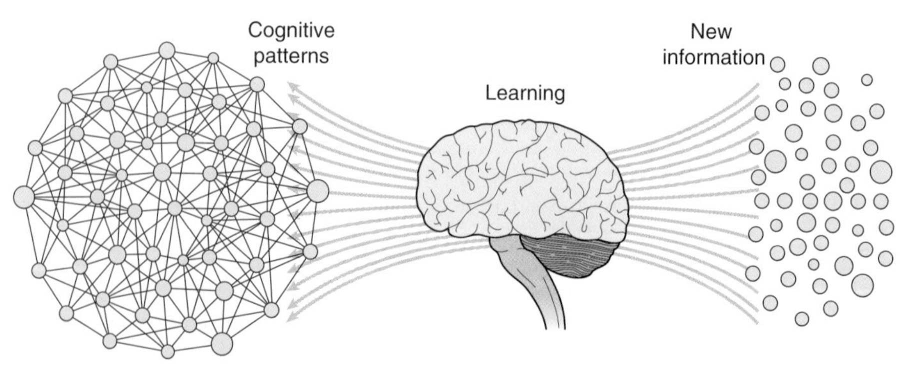

Fig. 5.7 Conceptual learning is characterized by patterns and multiple linkages. (Based on "Knowledge Information," Idiagram, © Marshall Clemens; available at http://www.idiagram.com/ideas/knowledge_integration.html.)

BOX 5.2 ■ Exemplar: Conceptual Learning in Action

Reyna, a nursing student, is learning about the concept of inflammation. Prior to the class, she read a chapter on the topic. In class she listened to a 15-minute presentation by the instructor and then viewed a 5-minute video highlighting the physiological response to inflammation. In her collaborative learning group, she shared a story about a time she experienced an inflammatory reaction and how her situation linked to what she just learned. Her group then completed a case study featuring a situation involving a patient with an inflammatory condition and reinforced risk factors, typical presentation, and collaborative interventions for the situation. The instructor led a discussion session about the case, posing specific questions to the learning groups, including the interrelationship of the concept of inflammation to other concepts. The class concluded with a short reflective writing activity in which Reyna wrote what she learned about her new understanding of the concept.

CONCEPTUAL APPROACH AND DEEP LEARNING

Conceptual learning encourages students to focus on big ideas (or concepts) and apply information or knowledge to specific situations for context. Learning complex subject matter, such as nursing and health care, requires the ability to transfer what has been previously learned into problem solving activities in the context of clinical situations. It does little good for students to learn about concepts in the absence of clinical examples, or exemplars. Benner and colleagues (2010) frame this from the position of integrative teaching practices—in other words, framing student learning of concepts and exemplars in the context of a patient situation or clinical problem. Conceptual learning, particularly when framed in a clinical context, engages the learner with an application of information to things that are clearly relevant. This engagement and active application of information facilitates understanding and commits this understanding to long-term memory (Box 5.2).

What Does All of This Mean for Nursing Faculty?

The preceding sections related to how the brain learns and conceptual learning underscore the need to rethink what is taught in nursing curricula and best practices for teaching. Superficial coverage of large volumes of nursing content must be replaced with a deep understanding of concepts. However, there must be a sufficient number of clinical examples (exemplars) to allow in-depth study; this is necessary to allow students to fully grasp the concept (Bransford et al., 2000). The use of relevant clinical exemplars is crucial for gaining a conceptual understanding. That said, faculty should frame the exemplar learning through the conceptual lens as opposed to learning about an exemplar with the concept as an after-thought. As an example, the exemplar heart failure should be taught through the lens of the concept of perfusion as opposed putting heart failure in the "center ring" with perfusion as the side show. Over time, the use of concepts to frame exemplars deepens conceptual understandings, thus making the case for an established set of concepts to be used over a curriculum.

TEACH WITH BALANCE

Traditionally, teaching has focused on delivering information in a student-passive approach. Assuming the students are paying attention, information is sent to the back portion of the cortex. The student must have an opportunity to integrate that information (using the frontal integrative cortex) to gain a deep and enduring understanding (Zull, 2002). Passive learning focusing on the memorization of facts is hard work because such an activity lacks context, and associations. It is just as problematic when students are exposed to learning activities without an infusion of information. Conceptual learning should be balanced with a focus on the concept. A combination of concrete experiences involving reflection and student-centered

MISCONCEPTIONS AND CLARIFICATIONS

Misconception: A student-centered learning activity is essentially the same as conceptual learning.

Clarification: Conceptual learning is enhanced with student-centered activities, but conceptual learning does not automatically occur simply by designing a student-centered learning activity. Optimal conceptual learning occurs when:

- Learners build on previous knowledge.
- The learning activity focuses on a concept and is tied to the clinical context.
- Students are fully engaged in the activity and perceive the learning activity as useful.
- Reflection is used to facilitate deep connections.
- The learning environment is safe.

learning where students are involved in abstract thought, problem solving asking questions (thinking), hands-on activities, and activities requiring students to test their assumptions are central to conceptual learning. The application of such cognitive skills leads to more effective learning.

PURPOSEFUL LEARNING

Conceptual learning must have a purpose that is apparent to the learner. Students' perception of the value of what is being learned influences motivation, which in turn influences what and how they learn (Ambrose et al., 2010). Transferring previous knowledge to a new learning situation is enhanced by not only creating a situation where students see the value or direct relationship to their area of study and the implications of why it is important, but that they can see the benefit while they are learning.

BUILD ON EXISTING KNOWLEDGE

Enhanced learning occurs when students can build on existing knowledge and apply new knowledge in purposeful ways. That the brain constructs new knowledge and understanding based on what a person already knows is an important principle that serves as a starting point for conceptual learning. It is also just as important for students to retrieve the necessary and appropriate knowledge to solve a problem. Preexisting knowledge should be considered as a starting point when creating conceptual learning activities. However, some learners have incomplete or inaccurate understandings, and this can interfere with new learning (Ambrose et al., 2010). For this reason, it is critical that learning be extended from a body of accurate information, which underscores the importance of assessing students' baseline understanding.

PURPOSEFUL REFLECTION

Reflecting on learning situations and experiences is one of the most important aspects of the conceptual approach and is a key to optimal learning in general. Reflection is a time to think about what has just happened in the learning situation and to actively contemplate things such as what was successful and what was not successful, how the situation differed from a previous situation, or how what was learned links to previously learned concepts. Faculty should build in reflection as part of conceptual teaching to optimize cognitive connections to concepts and clinical contexts.

MANAGE THE LEARNING ENVIRONMENT

Conceptual learning requires deep and purposeful thinking, and thus the learning environment must be free from unnecessary distractions and stress. Faculty must consider the tone of the classroom and the emotional state of students. For example, it is not uncommon for first-semester nursing students to feel completely overwhelmed with the nursing school experience. Added to that may be feelings of inadequacy in a highly competitive cohort, along with personal stressors. Collectively these things matter and can impair learning. Elimination of unnecessary emotional stressors in the classroom or curriculum and creating an emotionally secure environment (one where learners feel respected by their teachers and free from potentially embarrassing situations) helps to moderate other stressors.

EMOTION MATTERS

As in any learning situation, conceptual learning is optimized when learners are engaged and in a positive emotional state. Students do not typically become engaged when sitting and listening to a lecture. Therefore nursing faculty are encouraged to teach using a variety of conceptual strategies that enhance learner engagement in pleasurable ways. The real trick is learning to foster an emotional connection to material as opposed to just making learning fun. Novel teaching strategies that enhance curiosity are effective as long as there is actual learning involved. Concepts taught using unfolding case studies (featuring characters familiar to the students) or standardized patients enhance a positive emotional connection (Shuster, Giddens, & Roerigh, 2011).

Summary

Educational neuroscience refers to the science of learning and includes the interrelationship between neuroscience, teaching practices, and psychology. The brain processes associated with learning include sensing, integrating, and responding. The brain's ability to learn is impacted by multiple factors such as emotion, dopamine, sleep, nutrition, and movement. Best practices in education have shown that learning is most effective when students link to and apply previous knowledge to new situations. Conceptual learning directly applies such principles; students learn concepts as big ideas and apply these to multiple situations and contexts, resulting in neuroplasticity. Faculty can enhance conceptual learning by teaching with balance, managing the learning environment, creating emotionally engaging learning activities that are purposeful, and promoting focused reflection.

References

Ambrose S, Bridges M, Dipietro M, Lovett MC, Norman MK. *How Learning Works.* San Francisco, CA: Jossey-Bass; 2010.

Benner PB. *From Novice to Expert.* Menlo Park, CA: Addison Wesley; 1984.

Benner P, Sutphen M, Leonard V, et al. *Educating Nurses: A Call for Radical Transformation.* San Francisco, CA: Jossey-Bass; 2010.

Bransford JD, Brown AL, Cocking RR. *How People Learn: Brain, Mind, Experience, and School.* Washington, DC: National Academy Press; 2000.

Connell JD. The global aspects of brain-based learning. *Educational Horizons.* 2009;88:28–39.

Dragansk D, Gaser C. Neuroplasticity: changes in grey matter induced by training. *Nature.* 2004;427(22): 311–312.

Erikson HL, Lanning LA. *Transitioning to a Concept-Based Curriculum and Instruction.* Thousand Oaks, CA: Corwin Press; 2014.

Gee JP. *What Video Games Have to Teach Is About Learning and Literacy.* New York, NY: Palgrave Macmillan; 2007.

Jensen E. *Brain-Based Learning: The New Paradigm of Teaching*. 2nd ed. Thousand Oaks, CA: Corwin Press; 2008.

Kuypers L. *The Zones of Regulation*. http://www.zonesofregulation.com/index.html; 2017.

Shuster G, Giddens J, Roerigh N. Emotional connection and integration: dominant themes among undergraduate nursing students using a virtual community. *J Nurs Educ*. 2011;50:222–225.

Pawlak R, Magarinos AM, Melchor J, McEwen B, Strickland S. Tissue plasminogen activator in the amygdala is critical for stress-induced anxiety-like behavior. *Nat Neurosci*. 2003;6:168–174.

Salamone JD, Correa M. Motivational views of reinforcement: implications for understanding the behavior functions of nucleus accumbens dopamine. *Behav Brain Res*. 2002;137:3–25.

Sosa D. How science met pedagogy. In: Sosa D, ed. *Mind, Brain, and Education*. Bloomington, IL: Solution Tree Press; 2010.

Tanner CA. Thinking like a nurse: a research-based model of clinical judgment in nursing. *J Nurs Educ*. 2006;45(6):204–211.

Timpson WM, Bendel-Simso P. *Concepts and Choices: Meeting the Challenges in Higher Education*. Madison, WI: Magna Publications; 1996.

Willis J. The current impact of neuroscience on teaching and learning. In: Sosa D, ed. *Mind, Brain, and Education*. Bloomington, IL: Solution Tree Press; 2010.

Wolfson A, Carskadon M. Sleep schedules and daytime functioning in adolescents. *Child Dev*. 1998;69:875–887.

Zull JE. *The Art of the Changing Brain*. Sterling, VA: Stylus; 2002.

CHAPTER 6

Conceptual Teaching Strategies for the Classroom

Linda Caputi

This book has covered many aspects of the conceptual approach to nursing education. This chapter addresses implementation of a conceptual approach for teaching to enhance student learning. More specifically, this chapter provides an overview for conceptual teaching in a concept-based curriculum. Three common themes (the "3Cs") emerge from a larger view of this chapter: teaching the **C**oncept, developing **C**linical judgment, and using **C**ontext for meaningful learning. The 3Cs are useful as anchors to facilitate consistency in how concepts are taught. Because it is important to provide a theoretical basis for teaching, this chapter begins with a discussion about cognitive frameworks and teaching. The chapter then presents a discussion on developing and facilitating student thinking that leads to the type of thinking used in nursing practice. The last and largest part of the chapter presents how to develop a lesson plan for teaching a concept and how to effectively teach the concept by incorporating concept-based teaching strategies. Developing lesson plans is important for all learning environments—theory classroom, skills laboratory, simulation laboratory, and clinical. Conceptual teaching is implemented in all these learning environments.

Cognitive Frameworks

Constructivist learning theory explains the nature of learning as a process through which learners create their own learning. Constructivists believe information can be constructed in many different ways. As faculty introduce new information, students either add that new information to their existing cognitive frameworks or construct a new framework (Schunk, 2012). Cognitive frameworks, also known as *mental frameworks* and *schemata*, help the learner organize and interpret information and integrate new information with previously learned knowledge (Deane & Asselin, 2015). Cognitive frameworks can also be seen as a way of looking at the elements that provide a framework for the implementation of the teaching/learning process (Caputi, 2010). This is part of the *integrating process* discussed in Chapter 5 through which learners sort and group data and then make sense of those data, all of which occurs within their preexisting frameworks. The preexisting frameworks give meaning to incoming data. For example, when a nurse hears the phrase "2 by 4" or sees the notation "2×4," the nurse processes that information as meaning a type of wound dressing. However, a student with a different preexisting framework (a background in construction, as an example) may interpret that phrase in reference to a size of finished lumber. This different meaning may initially confuse the uninformed student when first encountering this information in a nursing context.

As learners build their cognitive frameworks in nursing, the process of integrating incoming information into an existing schema from a nursing perspective becomes automatic. Novices often do not have an established mental framework related to what they are learning in their nursing courses. The framework used by faculty to organize information has an impact on how students build cognitive frameworks in which to place and understand the information. A concept-based curriculum uses concepts as that framework.

LINEAR TEACHING AND COGNITIVE FRAMEWORKS

Nursing faculty have traditionally taught using a linear approach organized around specific content. For example, faculty teaching a medical condition in an adult-health nursing course often use a body systems/disease approach that looks similar to the method illustrated in Fig. 6.1.

In this example, the primary focus is on the health condition and is presented from the context of the primary body system affected. Anatomy, physiology, and pathophysiology are often discussed to frame the health condition and may be repetitive information from prerequisite courses. Each condition has a list of risk factors, signs and symptoms, and laboratory/diagnostic studies included with a discussion on assessment. Medical treatment and nursing management are discussed, along with expected patient outcomes. Throughout the course and other courses in the curriculum, other health conditions are organized in similar fashion, independent of each other, and often in the absence of a patient context or consideration of how the information applies to nursing practice. Subsequently, students memorize facts about each condition or content area and build discrete cognitive patterns that may look similar to those in Fig. 6.2. Organizing information into categories that are not within a patient context and are structured around diseases, with nursing interventions representing pieces of knowledge and information on the linear path, does little to provide relevance of the knowledge in practice situations. These frameworks are rather abstract, and students struggle to understand the relevance of all the parts (Benner, Sutphen, Leonard, & Day, 2010). Students often resort to using rote memorization of discrete and often disconnected information to learn. Furthermore, with such an approach faculty may miss key opportunities to connect the information to other important curriculum content such as safety, professionalism, quality improvement, and others. These topics are often taught in separate courses with the expectation that students will assemble this information in a meaningful way during their clinical experiences or simulation activities.

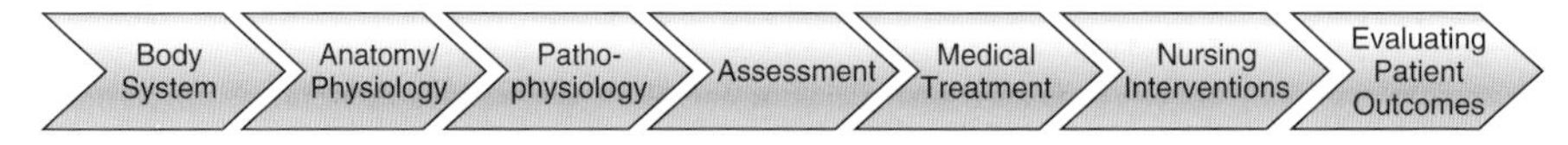

Fig. 6.1 Body Systems Model for teaching nursing content.

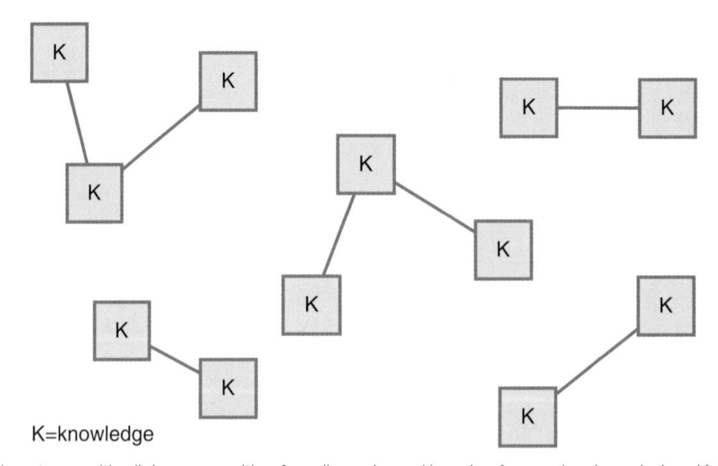

Fig. 6.2 Discrete cognitive linkages resulting from linear-based learning focused on knowledge. *K*, knowledge.

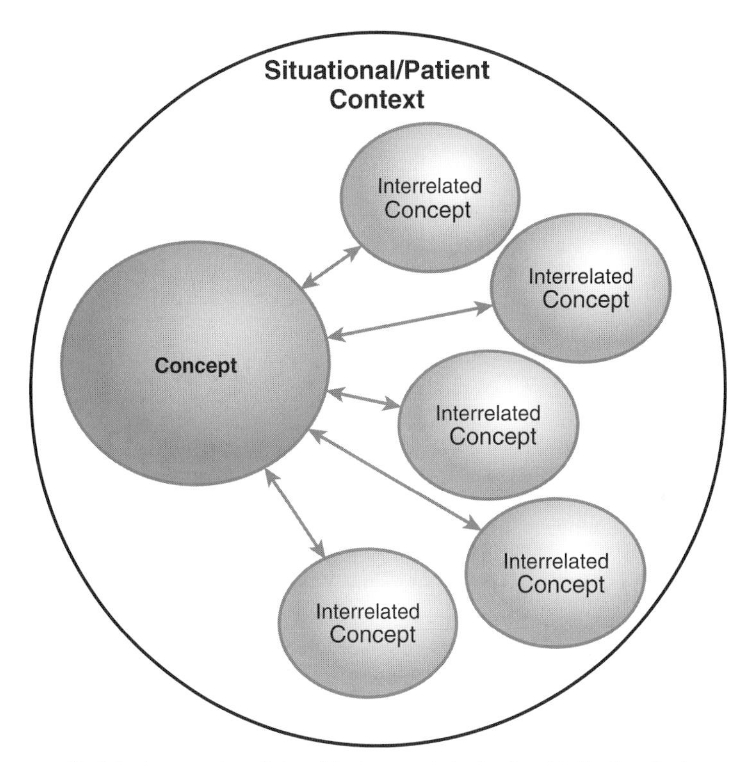

Fig. 6.3 A concept and interrelated concepts in situational/patient context.

CONCEPTUAL TEACHING AND COGNITIVE FRAMEWORKS

In the conceptual approach, faculty teach students about nursing by framing nursing content within concepts. Three categories of concepts previously described in Chapter 4 (Professional Nursing and Health Care Concepts, Health and Illness Concepts, and Health Care Recipient Concepts) are used as the basis to organize teaching and learning. Not only is the focus on specific concepts, but the student makes purposeful linkages to interrelated concepts within all three concept categories. Learning is nested in a situational context—that is, within the practice of nursing (Fig. 6.3).

Some of the same content taught in a traditional curriculum is still included in a concept-based curriculum, but much of the content is taught as concept exemplars rather than isolated health conditions within a body system approach. Teaching with a conceptual framework helps students develop cognitive patterns that look similar to those demonstrated in Fig. 6.4. These cognitive skills facilitate transferability of information to other concepts and is a necessary component to bridge students' thinking from a focus on content knowledge to the advancement to a conceptual level of understanding—or the ability to make generalizations.

COGNITIVE FRAMEWORKS AND HOW A NURSE THINKS

Let's take a closer look at how a nurse thinks when approaching a patient. The nurse's thinking may look something like that presented in Box 6.1. Although the experienced nurse has an

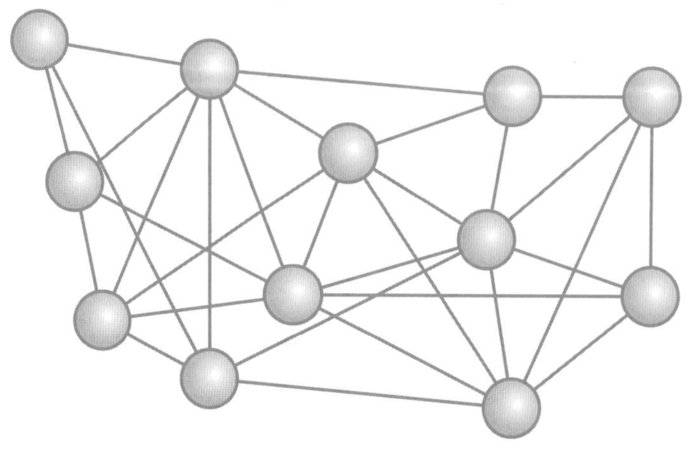

Fig. 6.4 Pattern recognition and cognitive linkages resulting from the conceptual approach.

BOX 6.1 ■ The Thinking Nurse

- Notice the patient's skin color and the concepts that skin color reflects (e.g., perfusion and oxygenation), which leads to an assessment of breathing characteristics and other related data; then consider laboratory test results, medications, and treatments related to these concepts.
- Consider how communication leads to an indication of cognition—the ability to process information. (Concept: Cognition)
- Consider anxiety and the concepts that anxiety reflects, such as pain, and then consider medication orders, treatments, and other concerns of the patient that may be causing the anxiety. (Concept: Anxiety)
- Consider safety as it relates to the environment. (Concept: Safety)
- Consider how tubes are related to hydration, output, and intravenous fluid orders. (Concept: Fluid balance)
- Consider care management or delegation.
- Consider how positioning is related to strength, mobility, and care management/delegation. (Concepts: Mobility; Care coordination)
- Consider how visitors interact and the patient's support system. (Concept: Family dynamics)
- Consider other concepts, such as culture and functioning ability.
- Consider the current and preexisting conditions and all the concepts that relate to these conditions.

expectation about how the patient will present based on the medical diagnosis, many other aspects of the patient's situation are assessed. According to Benner, Tanner, and Chesla (2009), the expert nurse has a deep understanding of the total situation and is able to focus immediately on salient aspects without wasting time and energy on a large range of alternative solutions. Thus the expert nurse takes in the whole picture of the patient.

Advanced thinking skills underlie the ability to make sound clinical judgments. The process of clinical judgment developed by Tanner (2006) was shown in Figure 1.3 in Chapter 1. According to Tanner, a nurse's response to a clinical situation is influenced by his or her knowledge, past experiences, and knowledge of the patient. This represents a baseline with regard to what the nurse expects to see and thus the ability to ***notice*** when patterns are inconsistent. Recognizing inconsistencies by applying a thorough understanding of each concept, the nurse gains additional information to correctly ***interpret*** the situation and ***respond*** appropriately. The actions taken during the respond step are dependent on the health care environment in which the nurse is working. The expert nurse then **reflects** on this experience, which further expands the nurse's knowledge and experience. The ability to make clinical judgments in this way is enhanced through conceptual thinking skills because of the cognitive connections students make when encountering new information. Reflective thinking, however, must be purposeful in this process for the base of knowledge and experience to grow (Tanner, 2006).

Thinking at a higher level is the topic of research by the National Council of State Boards of Nursing (NCSBN). The NCSBN is researching the use of alternate item types that represent much higher levels of thinking than measured with current items. This is a critical indicator of the need to focus nursing students on thinking as they are learning conceptually. The NCSBN also offers a research-based, clinical judgment model in nursing (Dickison, Luo, Woo, Muntean, & Bergstorm, 2016) that will serve as the basis for their measurement model used to develop questions that measure clinical judgment.

For these reasons, the students' method of learning should not be based on rote memorization but rather by making meaningful connections among concepts within the context of the patient and health care setting. Put another way, these relationships vary depending on the specific patient situation and the interrelated concepts involved. In fact, the medical condition may be near resolution and other issues may have developed that take priority. As an example, a patient might be experiencing anxiety associated with a pending discharge, family issues, or an array of other problems. Nurses identify and address these concerns and problems because these represent fundamental concepts associated with nursing practice, which is a broader perspective than simply focusing on a medical diagnosis.

Teaching students from a medical model approach results in a greater emphasis on disease management and does not emphasize concepts within a nursing framework. When students who have been taught using a medical model approach the patient, they often frame their assessment with an emphasis on signs and symptoms of the disease process as presented in their textbook. They might then evaluate the effect of treatments and look for evidence of complications. At some point in their practice, students must assume a different perspective (the patient's response to medical problems along with other health care concerns) to better position themselves to engage in nursing. For some, gaining this larger perspective may happen serendipitously or not at all.

Ideally, the patient's response to the medical problem is considered conceptually. The concepts addressed in Box 6.1 represent not only the patient's response to a medical problem but also the patient's response to many other health care issues. These findings represent the patient's responses, which are addressed by nurses. Many of these issues and concerns may be missed with a focus strictly on medical issues.

These considerations lead to the following questions: Would it not better serve students to teach them to think conceptually, using a concept-based cognitive framework rather than the medical model? If a concept-based cognitive framework is the focus of thinking that we want students to use, how do we teach this way of thinking? That is, the nurse assesses a patient and identifies an array of issues, concerns, and problems, in addition to those related to the medical diagnosis. Is this not the approach we aspire for students to use? It is critical that students be taught the concepts important to nursing practice and how they interrelate so they will be able to identify all patient concerns, regardless of their cause.

In a concept-based curriculum, the major nursing concepts are taught with a focus on application within nursing practice. Nursing program content is presented based on patient situations that launch a cascade of details about the concepts and related concepts, with health conditions and related problems the patient is experiencing just one piece of the total patient picture.

MISCONCEPTIONS AND CLARIFICATIONS

Misconception: An easy way to adapt a conceptual teaching approach is to use body systems as concepts, and then teach the same information using a similar manner as previously presented.

Clarification: Renaming body systems as concepts does not result in conceptual teaching because the emphasis is limited to a physiological/illness perspective. Although health and illness concepts relate to body systems (such as gas exchange, perfusion, nutrition, and others), many other concepts would not be included. The goal of concept-based teaching is for the learner to gain conceptual understanding. This requires a specific and purposeful approach to facilitate thinking by linking concepts to supporting content and the formation of generalizations.

Conceptual Teaching and Building Cognitive Connections

Nursing faculty must ensure that students learn how to use and apply information the way the nurse uses it—that is, the student learns to think like a nurse. In the content-focused, body-systems approach to teaching, the risk is great that students are expected to learn an excessive amount of information that grows larger each year with the expanding knowledge base of nursing. This plethora of information, which in the past has been determined to be essential for new nurses to learn, is overwhelming for students. Students tend to rely on memorization as the primary method of cognitive processing to meet their goal of passing the course. The problem with this approach is it is not representative of the way a nurse thinks in practice. Nurses do not spend their time merely recalling information, although recalling information is the first step. They must recall information, then use it in specific patient situations, or use the information to deal with a problem in the health care environment.

The overarching goal of conceptual teaching in nursing is to help learners build conceptual understandings of nursing that are transferable to a variety of patient and health care situations. It is an approach that emphasizes *learning the processes of thinking* rather than a focus on learning facts. A concept-based approach to teaching provides students with experience building on facts and connecting previous knowledge to develop cognitive patterns and using those patterns as a connection to new information. This is truly at the heart of conceptual learning. Faculty use a variety of teaching strategies that require students to look at nursing from the perspective of concepts important to nursing practice, coupled with active processing of information at the application and higher cognitive levels.

Building cognitive connections occurs when a student uses facts and previously learned information as a foundation when encountering new information. Recalling what was presented in Chapter 1, facts are bits of information that are specific and are embedded within topics or exemplars. Concepts are mental abstractions that frame a group of exemplars based on common attributes; concepts transcend time and situations. A concept is represented by multiple exemplars, and an exemplar can represent more than one concept. Understanding the connections of interrelated concepts leads to the ability to understand generalizations, principles, and theories.

Conceptual teaching encourages the student to learn how to recognize patterns and make connections, leading to deeper, transferable understandings (refer back to Fig. 6.4). Faculty should design teaching strategies that help students make sense of the factual knowledge and guide them to think intuitively on a higher level. This represents application of context while engaging in clinical judgment. Unfortunately, most nursing graduates are not able to think at the levels required in the current health care environment. In a recent study, Kavanagh and Szweda (2017) reported that only 23% of new graduate nurses think at the levels necessary for practice. This finding is down from the 34% reported by Del Bueno (2005) using the same research design with a sample of more than 5000 new graduates. Kavanagh and Szweda suggest a paradigm shift in the education of the next generation of nurses, which should include a comprehensive program-wide approach to teach students to think like a nurse.

Designing Concept-Based Learning Sessions for the Classroom

An important principle to remember is that teaching in a concept-based curriculum is not about teaching content related to a list of concepts; instead, the focus is on teaching for understanding and helping students learn to *think like a nurse* (Caputi, 2016). What does this mean? How do nursing faculty conduct a classroom session that results in students gaining a deep understanding of concepts? When teaching conceptually, keep these important principals in mind:

- Teach the concept! There should always be a formal concept overview or concept presentation for each concept in the curriculum.
- Teach designated exemplars for each concept.
- Link teaching to a patient or situational context.
- Link new information to preexisting understanding.
- Use a variety of student-centered teaching strategies for collaborative learning.

MISCONCEPTIONS AND CLARIFICATIONS

Misconception: Once a concept-based curriculum is in place, all faculty will automatically teach the curriculum in the way it was intended.

Clarification: Many faculty are comfortable teaching in the traditional manner and in a very linear fashion. Additionally, many students are comfortable with the traditional approach and may be resistant to concept-based, active learning strategies. These two factors often result in faculty teaching in the same manner as they always have rather than with a concept-based approach. Unfortunately, this results in a concept-based curriculum on paper but not in practice. Therefore evaluation data about the effectiveness of the concept-based curriculum are not reflective of a concept-based curriculum but of a traditional curriculum. It is important for faculty to teach the concept-based curriculum in the way it was intended, so evaluation data can accurately reflect the intent and effects of the concept-based curriculum.

TABLE 6.1 ■ **Concept Presentation Template for Health and Illness Concepts**

Topic	Description
Concept Definitions	A clear definition of the concept should be included so students (and faculty) are all working from a common definition; concept definitions can be easily found in the literature.
Scope or Categories of Concept	All concepts have scopes or categories; a scope is like a continuum (such as hyperthermia, normothermia, or hypothermia), whereas categories are discrete distinctions (such as types of infections).
Populations at Risk/Individual Risk Factors	Students should gain an understanding of what populations or individuals are most likely to have or to develop a problem with the concept, which is a critical skill for *noticing* as it relates to clinical judgment; help students differentiate populations at risk as opposed to individual risk factors.
Physiologic Processes and Consequences	Normal physiologic processes and the physiologic basis for dysfunction and consequences (i.e., what the individual experiences).
Assessment • History • Examination findings • Diagnostic tests	At the concept level, this section helps the student identify the individual's status as it relates to the concept (optimal functioning or dysfunction); again, this understanding is critical for clinical judgment.
Clinical Management • Primary prevention • Screening • Collaborative interventions	Students must gain a clear understanding of what they should do when encountering the health care recipient as it relates to the concept, which is also a critical element of clinical judgment; this comprehensive look at preventative, screening, or treatment options is performed to enhance or maintain optimal function or treat in situations of dysfunction and is not focused at the disease level but rather at the concept level; when exemplars are taught, the elements within this section should easily connect.
Interrelated Concepts	Students should consider how the concept links to other concepts; many concepts are closely interrelated (eg, perfusion and gas exchange); purposeful learning about these interrelationships establishes the cognitive patterns needed for making future connections.
Common Exemplars	Every concept has multiple exemplars although only a few are formally taught. Exemplars are taught by linking to the concept.

CONCEPT PRESENTATION

Each concept should be formally taught in depth (referred to as the *concept presentation).* The concept presentation should be incorporated within courses as part of curriculum planning. The sequencing of concept presentations is highly variable, depending on the curriculum design. Regardless of sequencing, faculty should develop a consistent approach to the concept presentation across all courses to enhance the development of students' expertise. Such a consistent approach is critical for curriculum integrity. A concept presentation includes many of the elements associated with a concept analysis, described in Chapter 3. The use of a standardized template to develop concept presentations is very helpful in achieving consistency. Table 6.1 is an example of a template that can be used to develop the concept presentation for Health and Illness Concepts. Table 6.2 is an example template for Professional Nursing and Heath Care Concepts or Health Care Recipient Concepts.

Once an outline of the concept presentation has been developed, faculty consider which learning activities to use for the concept presentation. As discussed in Chapter 5, learners benefit when a variety of teaching strategies is used. Developing a lesson plan for the concept presentation is helpful to create a balanced and purposeful learning experience for students. Table 6.3

TABLE 6.2 ■ **Concept Presentation Template for Professional Nursing and Health Care Concepts or Health Care Recipient Concepts**

Topic	Description
Concept Definitions	A clear definition of the concept should be included so students (and faulty) are all working from a common definition; concept definitions can be easily found in the literature.
Scope or Categories of Concept	All concepts have scopes or categories; a scope is like a continuum (such as novice to expert); categories are discrete distinctions (such as leadership styles).
Attributes	Attributes are the critical elements used to correctly identify the concept; they are like the "rule" for acceptance; attributes are essential for clarification related to recognition of the concept in practice.
Theoretical Links	Many of the professional nursing concepts and patient attribute concepts have strong links to a theory or theories, such as Tanner's Model of Clinical Judgment; students should gain a perspective about these theories to better understand the concept.
Context to Nursing and Health Care	The context to nursing and health care should help the student gain an understanding of the situational context in which the concept will be seen and how it applies to the practice.
Interrelated Concepts	Students should consider how the concept links to other concepts; many concepts are closely interrelated (e.g., quality and safety), and purposeful learning about these interrelationships establishes the cognitive patterns needed for making future connections.
Common Exemplars	Every concept has multiple exemplars although only a few are formally taught. Exemplars are taught by linking to the concept.

TABLE 6.3 ■ **Sample Lesson Plan for the Concept of Perfusion**

Focus Area	Teaching Strategies/Activities	Learning Outcome
Concept Introduction	• Instructor: Introduce concept definitions, categories (e.g., central perfusion and local perfusion) and scope (e.g., no perfusion, reduced perfusion, and optimal perfusion). • Learning Groups: Students share what they have previously learned or seen that links to perfusion categories and/or scopes.	Clearly articulates the concept
Concept Identification	• Instructor: Present populations at highest risk for perfusion problems; clarify how these are similar and different from individual risk factors. • Learning Groups: Students complete a table identifying common individual risk factors across the life span; groups report and the instructor clarifies answers. • Instructor: Present a profile of four persons; students identify individual risk factors for each person. • Instructor: Presentation/review focused on how perfusion can become impaired and physiological consequences with impairment; shows a short video that clearly illustrates this process. • Learning Groups: Students review assessment skills previously learned in their health assessment class and link data to central perfusion, local perfusion, or both. • Instructor: Show photos depicting clinical findings of impaired perfusion; the students describe the relevance of the signs. • Learning Groups: Students complete a worksheet on common diagnostic tests to evaluate perfusion (central and local).	Recognizes persons with optimal perfusion, those at risk, and those who are experiencing poor perfusion

Continued

TABLE 6.3 ■ **Sample Lesson Plan for the Concept of Perfusion—cont'd**

Focus Area	Teaching Strategies/Activities	Learning Outcome
Clinical Management	• Learning Groups: Assign half the groups to locate recommended health promotion strategies from Healthy People 2020 (each group has a different age group) and half the groups to locate recommended screening guidelines from the USPSTF (each group has a different age group); the groups report. • Instructor: Present lecture about clinical treatment guidelines for perfusion problems—procedures, surgical interventions, and pharmacotherapy.	Initiates appropriate interventions and assesses patient outcome
Transferable Ideas	• Learning Groups: Students will identify up to five curriculum concepts and draw a concept map showing interrelated connections. • Learning Groups: Students will brainstorm medical conditions they are aware of that represent perfusion problems and identify if it represents a central or peripheral perfusion problem; the instructor will clarify answers and add to lists generated for further consideration.	Application of principles to other concepts and clinical conditions
Notes	After the concept overview, the following exemplars will be used to deepen the students' understanding of perfusion: • Heart failure, • Acute myocardial infarction, • Peripheral vascular disease.	

USPSTF, U.S. Preventive Services Task Force.

shows an example of a lesson plan for a didactic classroom concept presentation for *Perfusion* and Table 6.4 shows an example of a lesson plan for a didactic classroom concept presentation for Health Promotion.

Similar planning should occur for all concepts. Notice that the sample lesson plans represent a balance between faculty-led and student-centered activities. The plans incorporate a situational context for learning enhancement and purposeful linkages to past learning that connects to the students' existing cognitive frameworks, which are critical elements to include in any lesson plan to enhance learning (Brown, Roediger, & McDaniel, 2014). Also note that the concept presentations do not include a presentation of exemplars, but students are encouraged to consider possible exemplars that link to the concept.

Purposeful connections to other concepts (in all three concept categories) are made as part of the lesson plan as well. One could make the case that all concepts connect to each other in some way, so the focus should be on the concepts that have the closest connection and greatest impact on the primary concept being discussed. As the interrelated concepts are discussed, the instructor asks the "So what?" question to establish the importance of knowing the typical interrelated concepts for a concept. The discussions should focus on the commonly associated interrelated concepts that comprise the enduring understandings about a concept that may apply to most patients or situations. Other interrelated concepts emerge when the concept is applied to a specific clinical context or specific patient situation. Another example of a learning activity related to interrelated concepts is presented later in this chapter.

TABLE 6.4 ■ **Sample Lesson Plan for the Concept Health Promotion**

Focus Area	Teaching Strategies/Activities	Learning Outcome
Concept Introduction	• **Individually/Pairs/Groups:** Write out one or two sentences of what the terms health promotion, health, wellness, and disease mean to you. Share your definitions with the person sitting next to you. Combine your ideas. Now find another group of two. As a group of four, share your ideas about these terms. Review definitions. How do your ideas link to the definitions you found? • **Instructor:** Share the World Health Organization definitions with the class; how are their definitions similar?	Student clearly articulates the meaning of the concept and related terms.
Scope of Concept	• **Instructor:** Show visual depiction of Primary, Secondary, and Tertiary Prevention. In discussion format, ask student for examples and differentiation of each. • **Instructor:** Show a visual depiction of the trajectory of health promotion (individual, family, community, etc.) as well as life span of individuals. Lead discussion regarding health promotion on these trajectories, noting obvious differences and similarities.	Articulates the three primary categories and application among various individuals and groups.
Concept Attributes	• **Instructor:** Review four attributes of health assessment—optimizes health, evidence-based, patient/family/community orientation, culturally relevant. • **Learning Groups:** Students review a common health promotion initiative (such as smoking cessation or breast feeding for infant health) and identify evidence of all attributes within the health initiative. • **Instructor:** Show slide of the WHO 12 Tips to Be Healthy and the 3 Pillars of Health Promotion. Discuss each of the slides in context of visibility within society, and challenges in implementation.	Recognizes consistent pillars and attributes present in all health assessment priorities.
Theoretical Links	• **Instructor:** Presents brief lecture on common health promotion models.	Attains a beginning-level awareness of how theory affects health promotion activities.
Nursing Role in Health Promotion	• **Instructor:** Lead discussion regarding differences in health promotion assessment between individual, family and community-based assessments. • **Learning Groups:** Students will complete jigsaw activity featuring the most common interventions to support health promotion and specific role of the nurse within these interventions.	Initiates appropriate interventions to achieve patient outcomes.
Transferable Ideas	• **Learning Groups:** Students will review an assigned health promotion policy. Using specific guidelines, they will determine how evidence, health disparities, patient education and health care economics apply to the assigned health promotion policy answers and add to lists generated for further consideration	Application of principles to other concepts and clinical conditions
Notes	After the concept overview, the following exemplars will be used to deepen the students' understanding of health promotion: • Physical activity, • Smoking cessation, • Blood pressure screening.	

TEACHING EXEMPLARS

After the concept presentation, exemplars are taught to give students an opportunity to understand the concept more deeply. An exemplar is an example of a health condition or situation in which the concept under study would be present. Faculty should teach the designated exemplars that best represent the concept (according to the curriculum plan) and resist the temptation to teach all exemplars from a previous curriculum. Teaching an excessive number of exemplars results in content saturation, with faculty reverting back to intense lectures and students engaging in rote memorization. This outcome minimizes the benefits of the concept-based approach (Giddens & Brady, 2007). Students will have opportunities to learn additional exemplars and to make linkages to concepts during clinical experiences.

When faculty teach the exemplar, purposeful linkages back to the concept presentation must be made. Faculty teach exemplars through the use of balanced teaching strategies and within the context of clinical practice. Exemplars provide a link to what students see in practice; they provide a link between content, the concept, and additional interrelated concepts specific to the exemplar.

Exemplars serve another purpose. Like all nursing knowledge, how concepts apply in practice depends on the situation. Concepts are usually altered and influenced by the context in which they are situated and are influenced by other factors relevant to a patient situation. Therefore exemplars presented in the context of a specific patient or practice situation provide an even deeper, more meaningful understanding of the concepts and enhance students' skill in knowledge transferability.

SITUATIONAL OR CONTEXTUAL TEACHING AND LEARNING

One of the traits of expert nursing faculty is integrated teaching—that is, framing what is being learned in a situational context (Benner et al, 2010). Situational or contextual learning helps students understand how the information they are learning is applied in practice, such as with a unique patient or professional nursing situation. "Putting new knowledge into a *larger context* helps learning" (Brown, Roediger, & McDaniel, 2014, p. 6). This type of contextual teaching enhances conceptual learning because it reinforces the purposefulness of the information and facilitates the learners' ability to transfer ideas from one situation to another.

Situational learning can be successfully applied in classroom settings in many other ways. One of the most commonly used methods is through the use of case studies. Case studies typically focus on a single situation relevant to the topic being studied, although an unfolding case study presents a situation over time. Another alternative is the use of "standardized virtual patients." Standardized virtual patients are fictional characters that support learning throughout a course or curriculum. Students become familiar with each standardized virtual patient (his or her health history, family situation, and living situation, for example), and faculty use these virtual patients on an ongoing basis for a number of learning activities. Several examples of the use of standardized virtual patients have been reported in the nursing literature (Croteau, Howe, Timmons, Nilson, & Parker 2011; Curran, Elfrink, & Mays, 2009; Giddens, 2007; Walsh, 2011). Box 6.2 presents an example of three fictitious families within a community. Each family member (character) has a brief profile that describes his or her current health condition. This example provides beginning variable information on three families. Faculty can enhance the information as needed to fit their needs. Faculty can then post the profiles of the characters in a course management system and then use these as a basis for evolving case studies throughout the curriculum.

BOX 6.2 ■ Example of Virtual Community Families

The Wright Family

- Jennifer, age 36 years, height 5′1″, weight 175 lb, works full time as an auditor for the state, volunteers for her children's activities.
- Alvin, age 41 years, height 5'9", weight 250 lb, works full time as a sales man, travels out of town 3 days a week, smokes 2 packs of cigarettes a day, takes medication for depression and hypertension, recently diagnosed with diabetes mellitus type 2.
- Michael, age 7 years, Jennifer's son from a previous marriage; easygoing personality, active in sports, good student, has exercise-induced asthma for 3 years, frequent upper respiratory tract infections in the winter.
- Oliva, age 2 years, Jennifer and Alvin's daughter. Attends day care, has frequent ear infections. Parents have difficulty controlling her temper tantrums.
- Frank, age 72 years, is Alvin's father. Lives in assisted living facility. Has mild dementia, frequent falls, osteoporosis, severe emphysema (smoker for 60 years). Broke hip last year; currently uses a walker.

The Hernandez Family

- Juliette, age 43 years, height 5′4″; weight 150 lb, in good health but frequently has back pain. Works two jobs (waitress and cleaning offices). Five children ages 27, 25, 23, 18, and 15 years—the youngest two still live in the home.
- Julio, age 45 years, height 5′7″ weight 130 lb, in good health. Works on a construction crew as a dry wall installer; smokes one pack of cigarettes per day and drinks 3 to 6 beers daily. Speaks fluent Spanish, and some English. Grew up in Mexico, has been in United States since age 18. Parents and 3 sisters remain in Mexico, visits them periodically.
- Alberto, age 18 years, in good health. Attends the local community college and works part-time with Julio on construction crew. Fluent in Spanish, and English. Smokes cigarettes and marijuana; volunteers to help neighborhood children learn English.
- Katie, age 15 years, in good health. Had a recent miscarriage but did not tell her family. Excellent student (earns A's in school), has a steady boyfriend who is occasionally physically abusive.
- Several times a year two to three relatives or friends of relatives from Mexico stay with the Hernandez family in hopes of finding a job and permanent place to live.

The Warner Family

- Josephina, African-American, age 37 years, height 5′4″ weight 135 lb, in good health except for uterine fibroid disease. Is a lawyer, has one child living at home.
- Daniel, African-American, age 45 years, height 6′3″ weight 215 lb. Works in technology, internet security industry. Former football player, has frequent joint pain in knees, hips, back. Has type 2 diabetes (for 6 years) and diagnosed with hypertension four 4 years ago.
- Ethan, African-American, age 18 years, height 6′1″ weight 190 lb, a senior at a private high school. Excellent student, plays on the basketball team and is a member of the orchestra. Is considering options for college. Although some of his friends use drugs, Ethan does not.
- Dolly, African-American, age 70 (Daniel's mother) lives in a Memory Care center near their home. Has Alzheimer's disease, type 2 diabetes, chronic obstructive pulmonary disease (40 pack-year smoking history), myocardial infraction 2 years ago, and heart failure.

LINK TO PREEXISTING UNDERSTANDING

As discussed at the beginning of the chapter, faculty can facilitate conceptual learning by providing opportunities for students to construct new knowledge from previous understanding. A teaching strategy that faculty can use to determine students' preexisting understanding about a concept is to engage students in reflective thinking and guided discussion. Students are provided guided questions or a worksheet to complete either as a pre-class assignment or an in-class discussion activity. The questions and activities on the worksheet depend on the concept and the information you wish the students to recall from prior learning. Another approach that can be used to explore the students' preexisting understanding about the concept is a short questionnaire administered at the beginning of the class (Hardin & Richardson, 2012). Faculty can correct students' misconceptions or acknowledge their understandings about a concept as they discuss the concept in a non-nursing context. The concept is then taught in a nursing context when the concept may take on a different meaning or different application. Just as the meaning of a word takes on different meanings when used in different contexts, so will the meaning of nursing concepts. For example, the concept of *Family Dynamics* may take on a different meaning apart from the meaning used in a nursing context.

As the student progresses through the nursing program, the meaning of any one concept may expand as it is applied to different populations and settings as well as to increasingly complex situations. It may be difficult for students to shift their ideas about concepts, especially some that are deeply engrained in their belief systems. Concepts related to belief systems can be difficult to unlearn (Hardin & Richardson, 2012). However, identifying and clarifying misconceptions is an important element in helping students to think like a nurse. Active, meaningful learning across the curriculum with multiple exposures to the concept used in nursing is required to enable students to apply the concept from a nursing perspective.

TEACHING STRATEGIES FOR COLLABORATIVE, STUDENT-CENTERED LEARNING

As mentioned throughout this book, the instructor must abandon teaching practices that emphasize content and facts and adopt student-centered approaches that require active application or analysis of information, thus linking learning to concepts within the context of nursing practice.

There are a large number of teaching strategies that can be used to promote student-centered conceptual learning (Box 6.3). However, it is not the teaching strategy itself that makes it a concept-based teaching strategy. Conceptual teaching incorporates a number of teaching strategies focused on a concept—and the emphasis on conceptual understanding. The teaching strategy

BOX 6.3 ■ Teaching Strategies That Support Conceptual Learning

- Simulation
- Traditional Case Study
- Unfolding Case Study
- Virtual Communities
- Gaming
- Jigsaw
- Debate
- Guided Questions
- Concept assessment
- Risk Factor Assessment
- Pair and Share Discussions
- Compare and Contrast
- Vignettes
- Audiovisual (videos, songs)
- Storytelling
- Role Play
- Concept Analysis
- Concept maps
- Case writing
- Classroom response systems

BOX 6.4 ■ Helpful Tips for Teaching Conceptually

1. The focus of teaching and learning should be primarily on the concept. Exemplars are used to enhance the students' understanding of the concept and within the context of health care.
2. Prepare a concept presentation using a standardized concept-presentation format to enhance consistency for students.
3. Teaching should incorporate the 3 Cs: concept, critical thinking, and context whenever possible or as appropriate.
4. Consider the lesson objectives/course learning outcomes, and engage students at that level. Be aware of the type of thinking required to complete the in-class activities.
5. Prepare a lesson plan for each concept. Consider using a standardized template for each concept lesson plan (see Tables 6.3 and 6.4). Lesson plans should include:
   - pre-class assignments
   - in-class teaching strategies should include a combination of instructor-lead and student-centered approaches that require application of information. A significant amount of planned time in class should be devoted to active learning in small groups.
6. Faculty facilitate learning of students in collaborative learning environment by augmenting and enhancing information. Ask guiding questions to extend thinking further.

should help students construct a cognitive framework based on concepts, and thus concepts are the unifying, driving focus of the teaching techniques. Learning activities should actively engage students, focus on a clinical situation, require students to think, and be meaningful. Students should clearly understand how the activity contributes to their learning.

Faculty are often reluctant to have students work in learning groups for fear students may not participate or lack the ability to complete the work correctly. The power of collaborative learning is that students engage on a different level than they do when listening to a lecture. When students work in teams, the combined effect of different brains thinking together—particularly if they are encouraged to look for information online or in their textbook—typically results in accurate work. The role of the faculty member, as the facilitator of learning, is to provide guidance as students complete the activities and to redirect if students are arriving at incorrect conclusions. Short collaborative learning activities integrated within faculty-led discussions (as shown in Tables 6.3 and 6.4) are very effective for various aspects of the concept or exemplar presentations. This section presents several examples of strategies that can be applied to various aspects of concept or exemplar learning as individual or collaborative learning activities. Box 6.4 presents helpful tips for teaching conceptually.

Guided Questions

Guided questions are an effective teaching strategy that can be used with any part of a concept presentation. This teaching strategy gives students the opportunity to actively engage in thinking about the concept and what it means to them. Guided questions encourage students to connect what they already know to the new information they are learning. This also provides faculty with valuable information about the students' current understanding of the topic and how to direct the classroom discussion. Box 6.5 presents an example of guided questions used in a concept introduction of Collaboration.

BOX 6.5 ■ Example of Guided Discussion Questions for the Concept of Collaboration

1. Based on your readings and/or previous experiences, what does the word "collaborate" mean to you?
2. Describe a situation in which you experienced effective or successful collaboration with others. Why was the collaboration effective or successful?
3. Describe a situation in which you experienced ineffective or unsuccessful collaboration with others. Why was it unsuccessful?

Drawing on Past Experiences

All students have previous experiences or are aware of the experiences of others. Use past experiences to bridge students' thinking to new situations. Table 6.5 provides an example of a collaborative in-class learning activity that directs students to discuss the various dimensions of motivation in the context of health care management, based on past experiences they have seen or heard about. In this specific example, the learning activity helps students learn about the scope or categories of the concept, as part of the concept overview.

Risk Factor Assessment

Table 6.6 provides an example of a collaborative in-class learning activity for thermoregulation. In this activity, students consider why age groups have different risks for problems associated with thermoregulation. This collaborative work is assigned as an alternative to having an instructor present a slide listing risk factors. Alternatively, completion of this table may be used as a pre-class assignment. In class students can work in groups to compare and contrast and then develop a final table for presentation to the class.

TABLE 6.5 ■ **Example of a Teaching Strategy: Scope of Motivation as a Concept**

In your learning groups, share examples or situations in health care management you have seen or heard about that illustrate the concept of *Motivation* across the trajectory of no motivation to intrinsic motivation.

Level of Motivation	Example or Situation
Intrinsic *Motivation*	
Extrinsic *Motivation* with self-determination	
Extrinsic *Motivation* without self-determination	
No *Motivation*	

TABLE 6.6 ■ **Example of a Teaching Strategy: Risk Factor Assessment for the Concept of Thermoregulation**

In your learning groups, identify common risk factors for thermoregulation problems across the life span.

Infants & Children	Adolescents/ Young Adults	Older adults	Conclusion: How are risk factors similar? How are they different?

Adapted from TEACH for nurses for Giddens JF. *Concepts for Nursing Practice.* 2nd ed. St. Louis, MO: Elsevier; 2017.

Poster Fair

A variation on student presentations is the poster fair, a collaborative learning activity where student groups prepare and present posters to other members of the class. Box 6.6 shows an example of a poster fair as a learning activity for the concept of *Health Promotion* with a focus on interventions. Specifically, in this case student groups prepare posters for an in-class poster health fair outlining the current evidence for health promotion and health screening for various topics. Students learn from each other about the topics rather than from a faculty-driven presentation.

Concept Exemplars

Table 6.7 presents an example of a collaborative in-class learning activity in which students access the website of the Centers for Disease Control and Prevention to determine the most common types of infections in the United States (or their state) by age group. This activity links to the concept presentation and helps students gain an awareness of the broad range of exemplars they are likely to encounter in clinical practice. It is again important to reinforce the fact that instructors will not be teaching all the exemplars listed.

Concept Maps

Student-developed concept maps provide a window into the mind of the student as he or she diagrams how concepts interrelate (Caputi & Blach, 2008). Students work in pairs or small groups to first develop simple maps and then expand those maps to demonstrate a growing complexity of

BOX 6.6 ■ Collaborative Learning Activity for Health Promotion

In your learning groups, you will create a poster highlighting current evidence-based recommendations for your assigned health promotion topic. Be sure to include the parameters of the guidelines, particularly for specified population groups or persons with known risk factors, as appropriate. Include your reference. After groups have developed their posters, a poster fair will be held, and each group will share with others the key points for their topics.

TABLE 6.7 ■ Example of a Teaching Strategy: Identifying Common Exemplars for the Concept of Infection by Age Group

In your learning groups, visit the website of the Centers for Disease Control and Prevention and identify the 10 most common reported infections by age group.

Infants & Children	Adolescents/Young adults	Older adults	Conclusions: How are these similar and different?
1.	1.	1.	
2.	2.	2.	
3.	3.	3.	
4.	4.	4.	
5.	5.	5.	
6.	6.	6.	
7.	7.	7.	
8.	8.	8.	
9.	9.	9.	
10.	10.	10.	

Adapted from TEACH for nurses for Giddens JF. *Concepts for Nursing Practice.* 2nd ed. St. Louis, MO: Elsevier; 2017.

BOX 6.7 ■ Collaborative Learning Activity for Development and Interrelated Concepts

Consider the following concepts previously learned in your courses:

- *Culture*
- *Family Dynamics*
- *Genetics*
- *Nutrition*
- *Sensory Perception*

In your learning groups, discuss the relationship of these concepts to the concept of *Development*. Draw a concept map showing the relationships.

TABLE 6.8 ■ **Example of a Teaching Strategy: Compare and Contrast Degrees of Immunity**

As a group activity, students create a list of common symptoms and clinical findings associated with suppressed and exaggerated immunity and then discuss why each symptom or clinical finding occurs from a physiologic perspective.

Common clinical findings: Suppressed immunity	Common clinical findings: Exaggerated immunity

Adapted from TEACH for nurses for Giddens JF. *Concepts for Nursing Practice.* 2nd ed. St. Louis, MO: Elsevier; 2017.

concepts throughout the curriculum. For example, students work individually or in small groups to develop a concept map showing the relationship between *Development* and other concepts learned in the curriculum (Box 6.7). Students then discuss their rationale for the relationships made.

Compare and Contrast

An excellent teaching strategy to promote thinking is comparing and contrasting similar situations or opposite ends of a spectrum. This technique can be used as an in-class collaborative learning activity, or students can complete the task independently, after which the results can be used as discussion points in class. Table 6.8 provides an example of comparing and contrasting suppressed and exaggerated immune responses. Once the table is discussed, the information should be applied in class to several patient situations. The compare-and-contrast technique can be used for a number of different concepts in many different ways. As another example, compare and contrast can be used to highlight similarities and differences in a concept or exemplar based on age. Students are asked to compare and contrast the exemplar of asthma in a 70-year-old man and an 8-year-old girl. Such an activity not only provides an opportunity to gain a deeper understanding of the concept of gas exchange, but also to gain an understanding of the variation in how the exemplar presents in different situations and the unique interrelated concepts for each of the two cases.

Questions That Promote Thinking

Faculty can challenge students to apply their thinking by presenting questions in the classroom for students to answer. Typically this activity is performed using an audience response system. Once students have considered the question, before providing the answer, ask students to discuss their answers with a fellow student who answered differently. The students should discuss their answers and the rationales for their answers. They will either convince their peer to change his or her answer or change their own answer based on new insights. Students engage in deep, meaningful learning as they are discussing their thinking processes with their peers. Of course, to be a conceptual learning method, the questions must be focused on concepts and not bits of information about the topic (Hardin & Richardson, 2012).

DEVELOPING ENDURING UNDERSTANDINGS AND METACOGNITION

A primary purpose of active learning strategies that focus on concepts is to build enduring understandings—that is, discovering the concepts that interrelate and their enduring relationships across populations, health conditions, and health care settings. Students must be taught to think so they can develop enduring understandings. The active learning strategies described in this chapter guide students through the thinking process. By engaging in these activities, they are not just learning information but are gaining insight into the way a nurse thinks. Guided thinking activities in the context of the concepts help students develop their metacognitive skills, which is the ability to understand and monitor their own thinking. Metacognition is a critical skill for nursing students to practice. The goal of developing metacognition is achieved by making the learning process explicit with regard to learning how to think. The volume of information nurses must process each day requires learning how to approach thinking so the information becomes meaningful and endures across patient populations. A systematic, formal process to teach students thinking throughout the nursing program facilitates the formation of clinical judgment (Caputi, 2016; Caputi, 2018; McNelis, Ironside, Ebright, Dreifuerst, Zvonar, & Conner, 2014).

Summary

Teaching conceptually requires a purposeful process to involve students in learning experiences that help them develop thinking skills that advance their ability to build a web of cognitive connections through conceptual understandings within the discipline of nursing. Developing a deep understanding of concepts requires the construction of cognitive frameworks through the lens of how nurses think. Purposeful, planned learning sessions for each concept in the curriculum is needed. The use of a standardized approach and the incorporation of the three Cs (concepts, clinical judgment, context) underlie successful approaches to conceptual teaching. As evidenced by the variety of teaching strategies presented in this chapter, many teaching methods are used in a concept-based curriculum. Although only a sample of examples are presented, the underlying principles are that learning activities are deliberately planned with concepts being the major organizing factor, that the learning activities build on previous learning, and that learning is student centered.

References

Benner P, Sutphen M, Leonard V, Day L. *Educating Nurses: A Call for Radical Transformation.* San Francisco, CA: Jossey-Bass; 2010.

Benner P, Tanner C, Chesla C. *Expertise in Nursing Practice: Caring, Clinical Judgment, and Ethics.* 2nd ed. New York, NY: Springer; 2009.

Brown PC, Roediger HL, McDaniel MA. *Make It Stick: The Science of Successful Learning*. Cambridge, MA: The Belknap Press of Harvard University Press; 2014.

Caputi L, Blach D. *Teaching Nursing Using Concept Maps*. Glen Ellyn, IL: DuPage Press; 2008.

Caputi L. The Caputi model for teaching thinking in nursing. In: Caputi L, ed. *Innovations in Nursing Education*. vol. 3. Philadelphia: Wolters Kluwer; 2016:3–12.

Caputi L. *Think Like a Nurse: A Handbook*. Rolling Meadows, IL: Windy City Publishers; 2018.

Caputi L. An overview of the education process. In: Caputi L, ed. *Teaching Nursing the Art and Science*. 2nd ed. vol. 1. Glen Ellyn IL: DuPage Press; 2010:27–47.

Croteau SD, Howe LA, Timmons SM, Nilson L, Parker VG. Evaluation of the effectiveness of "The Village": a pharmacology education teaching strategy. *Nurs Educ Perspect*. 2011;32(5):338–341.

Curran R, Elfrink V, Mays B. Building a virtual community for nursing education: the town of Mirror Lake. *J Nurs Educ*. 2009;48(1):30–35.

Deane WH, Asselin M. Transitioning to concept-based teaching: a discussion of strategies and the use of Bridges change model. *J Nurs Educ Pract*. 2015;5(10):52–59.

DelBueno D. A crisis in critical thinking. *Nurs Educ Perspect*. 2005;26(5):278–282.

Dickison P, Luo X, Kim D, Woo A, Muntean W, Bergstrom B. Assessing higher order cognitive constructs by using an information-processing framework. *Journal of Applied Testing Technology*. 2016;17(1):1–19.

Giddens JF, Brady DP. Rescuing nursing education from content saturation: the case for a concept-based curriculum. *J Nurs Educ*. 2007;46(2):65–69.

Giddens JF. The neighborhood: a web-based platform to support conceptual teaching and learning. *Nurs Educ Perspect*. 2007;28(5):251–256.

Hardin PK, Richardson SJ. Teaching the concept curricula: theory and method. *J Nurs Educ*. 2012;51(3):155–159.

Kavanagh JM, Szweda C. A crisis in competency: the strategic and ethical imperative to assessing new graduate nurses' clinical reasoning. *Nurs Educ Perspect*. 2017;38(2):57–62.

McNelis AM, Ironside PM, Ebright PR, Dreifuerst KT, Zvonar SE, Conner SC. Learning nursing practice: a multisite, multimethod investigation of clinical education. *J Nurs Regul*. 2014;4(4):30–35.

Schunk DH. *Learning Theories: An Educational Perspective*. 6th ed. Upper Saddle River, NJ: Pearson; 2012.

Walsh M. Narrative pedagogy and simulation: future directions for nursing education. *Nurse Educ Pract*. 2011;11:216–219.

Tanner CA. Thinking like a nurse: a reserach model of clinical judgement in nursing. *J Nurs Edu*. 2006;45(6):204–211.

CHAPTER 7

Conceptual Teaching Strategies for Clinical Education

Jean Giddens ■ Linda Caputi

Clinical teaching and learning represents an important component of nursing education by enabling students to apply knowledge, concepts, and clinical skills learned in the classroom to the practice setting. Clinical learning activities provide the opportunity to extend and deepen students' conceptual understandings because they directly experience concepts associated with the nursing discipline as they appear in practice. Because of the complexity of health care, astute students will quickly notice that concepts take on a multitude of variations across clinical practice areas and across a variety of patients; this awareness is critical for developing more complex cognitive patterns of thinking that lead to clinical judgment. However, being in a clinical setting does not automatically result in deepened conceptual understandings; clinical education must be intentionally designed to achieve this outcome. This chapter provides an overview of planning and implementing conceptual teaching strategies in the clinical setting.

Traditional Clinical Education

The primary learning activity in a traditional clinical education model is for nursing students to provide total patient care to an assigned patient (or patients) in parallel with nursing staff. The traditional model is instructor-centered and further characterized by independent student learning with an emphasis on skills, extensive preclinical paperwork, extensive written assignments (care plans) to be submitted after clinical, and a disconnect between clinical learning and learning in didactic courses. The sustainability of this model, which has been the standard for more than 50 years (despite changes to education and health care), has largely been based on the assumption that learning occurs as a result of performing that care. However, the effectiveness of this model has come into question and is no longer considered an effective way for students to learn how to provide safe, quality nursing care that improves patient outcomes (Institute of Medicine [IOM], 2010; Tanner, 2010). For one thing it is difficult for the clinical instructor to effectively facilitate learning with a large group of students who are all providing total patient care. Also, the type of learning experiences students gain is dependent on patient acuity and the times students are in the clinical setting. Furthermore, the presence of multiple students simultaneously performing total patient care places an unnecessary burden on nursing staff within the clinical area. Traditional clinical education has been described as "education by random opportunity" (LeFlore, Anderson, Michael, Engle, & Anderson, 2007, p. 170)—underscoring the point that it represents limited consistency. Because typical activities of students are directed at patient care, this model essentially misplaces the student in the role of a nurse as opposed to the role of learner.

In a study evaluating outcomes associated with traditional clinical education, researchers reported that 1) students had too much "down time"; 2) too much time was focused on performing repetitive tasks that do not result in new learning; and 3) too little time was focused on developing higher-order thinking skills (Ironside & McNelis, 2010). In a subsequent study, McNelis and colleagues reported that higher level thinking was not a primary focus in pre-licensed nursing clinical education and that thinking at the application and analysis level was not rewarded (McNelis, Ironside, Ebright, Dreifuerst, Zvonar & Conner, 2014). Although students spend a large amount of time in the clinical setting, many of those clinical hours fail to result in productive learning. Faculty report spending most of their time supervising students in hands-on procedures, leaving little time to focus on fostering the development of clinical reasoning skills (IOM, 2010; McNelis, et al., 2014). It was pointed out more than a decade ago that "not all learning objectives require students to practice total patient care" (Gaberson & Oermann, 2007, p. 95). Moreover, not everything that needs to be learned can be effectively accomplished when providing total patient care. Although still prevalent, traditional approaches are slowly giving way to more contemporary clinical education practices.

Fundamentals of Contemporary Clinical Nursing Education and Conceptual Learning

New trends in clinical education have emerged to better prepare students for entry-level clinical practice. Contemporary clinical education approaches align with the clinical learning that is essential and desired in a concept-based curriculum. In the clinical setting, concepts come alive through a multitude of situations and activities. Clinical experiences serve as additional exemplars on which to extend and deepen conceptual understandings. Competencies associated with selected concepts can be used as measurable clinical outcomes associated with clinical education and practice. Advocates for changes to clinical education emphasize the need for deepening understanding of key concepts and application of thinking to develop clinical judgement (Caputi, 2018; Oermann, Shellenbarger, Gaberson, 2018; Giddens & Brady, 2007; Jessee, 2018; Lasater & Nielsen, 2009a; Nielsen, 2016; Tanner, 2006). Contemporary clinical education allows students to gain a deep understanding of concepts through the interaction and application in a clinical context. Tanner (2010) proposed three foci for clinical education to better prepare students for safe practice: 1) Deepening and extending theoretical knowledge and learning how key concepts are exemplified in practice; 2) Developing clinical judgment using a variety of thinking skills and strategies; and 3) Developing an understanding of the culture of health care and nursing and how the health care system functions, especially as it relates to the patient, the nurse, and interactions with other interprofessional health care providers. Thus the contemporary model of education not only supports conceptual learning but also supports student-centered learning with an emphasis on communication, collaboration, peer or group learning, and the development of clinical reasoning and clinical judgement.

OUTCOMES OF CONCEPT-BASED CLINICAL EDUCATION

Schools that adopt a concept-based curriculum share a similar perspective regarding the approach for education. Several contextual factors that influence decisions made within each program (such as type of nursing program, setting of the program, and resources) make each curriculum unique—thus faculty must make decisions about the approach for clinical education that aligns with the curriculum. Although the clinical education plan is driven by unique curriculum outcomes, the three learning domains—cognitive, psychomotor, and affective—underlie learning outcomes and are foundational to conceptual learning activities. Focus areas for each domain in clinical teaching are presented in Table 7.1. Faculty should consider these domains as a key part of the overall clinical education design.

Table 7.1 ■ **Domains of Learning and Focus Areas in Clinical Education**

Cognitive Domain	Psychomotor Domain	Affective Domain
• Problem Solving • Critical Thinking • Clinical Judgment & Decision Making	• Psychomotor Skills • Interpersonal Skills • Organizational Skills	• Professional Roles • Accountability • Ethics • Values

CLINICAL LEARNING SITES

Another key element that differentiates contemporary clinical education models from the traditional model is the use of a variety of settings for clinical learning. In a traditional setting, a nursing faculty member has a group of nursing students typically within an inpatient unit. This setting remains an important component of clinical education. However, as the role of professional nursing has evolved, so too has the setting where professional practice occurs; clinical education should incorporate diverse and non-traditional settings into the clinical education plan. As Oermann, Shellenbarger, Gaberson, (2018) point out, "nursing care can be learned wherever students have contact with patients" (p. 35). Many other common patient care areas (such as outpatient clinics, perioperative settings, nursing homes, extended care facilities, and hospice and palliative care settings) tend to be underused for clinical teaching. The evolution of contemporary clinical education has led to the expansion of clinical learning to diverse sites within the community (such as childcare and early education program, schools, summer camps, wellness centers) and international opportunities (Oermann, et al.). In addition to these patient care sites, the clinical laboratory and simulation laboratory have become increasingly prevalent for clinical education. Concept-based clinical learning experiences can easily be designed to occur in all clinical settings described, with an emphasis on learning within the context of the clinical site and with patients typically associated within the site. Nurse educators must be willing to reimagine clinical education to optimize this opportunity.

Obviously, clinical sites must provide the ability for students to meet the learning outcomes of the course. The type of patients seen and care provided within the site are two important factors. A positive environment that is inviting to students and committed to support student learning is just as important. Nurses at at the clinical site are integral to the students' learning, thus gaining their support and cooperation is essential. Inpatient units accustomed to supporting the learning of students in a traditional clinical education model may need additional reinforcement of the learning to take place to avoid confusion and facilitate cooperation.

TYPES OF CLINICAL LEARNING ACTIVITIES

Conceptual learning in the clinical setting is achieved through a variety of learning experiences and settings. A combination of *total patient care activities (TPCAs)* and *focused clinical learning activities (FCLAs)* with an intentional focus on concepts that foster the development of thinking and clinical judgement are used to optimize learning. The Oregon Consortium for Nursing Education was an early proponent of purposefully embedding a variety of structured clinical learning experiences (including direct clinical care experiences, concept-based experiences, case-based experiences, skill-based experiences, and integrative experiences) into a curriculum model (Gubrud-Howe & Schoessler, 2008).

Total Patient Care Activities

A TPCA refers to a clinical assignment where the student is responsible for planning, implementing, and evaluating care for one or more patients. This type of learning requires the students to integrate multiple aspects of care into the clinical experience and demonstrate of competence in patient care management. The instructor determines what the level of care interventions the student will do during total patient care activities; this is largely driven by care practices in the clinical site, and level of student. Variations of TPCAs include assigning more than one patient to a student or assigning one or more patients to more than one student (student teams). TPCAs typically occur in inpatient units but can also occur in outpatient areas and in simulation laboratory settings. In a concept-based curriculum, the application of concepts are incorporated into TPCAs through written assignments, discussions with the faculty member, and in clinical conference.

Focused Clinical Learning Activities

A FCLA (also referred to as a *focused concept learning activity*) is a structured learning experience designed to support various aspects of clinical learning to fulfill specific course or program learning outcomes. In a concept-based curriculum, the focus of learning is based on one or more concepts in a specific clinical context (Nielsen, 2009). For example, a FCLA could feature the concept of *Infection.* Depending on the design, FCLAs can be completed by students independently or in groups in any clinical learning setting. Most FCLAs involve direct interaction with patients; however, some involve indirect or limited patient interactions to accomplish the clinical learning objective. For example, a FCLA may focus on an observation experience involving communication patterns among health professionals, or another may focus on one aspect of nursing leadership or management. Shadowing and observational experiences are opportunities to develop a greater understanding of concepts associated with professional nursing practice, and interprofessional practice.

DESIGNING CONCEPT-BASED CLINICAL LEARNING ACTIVITIES

As discussed previously, contemporary clinical education is intentionally planned as part of the overall curriculum design by considering the learning outcomes, the desired learning domains, desired concepts, the level of the learner, and setting where clinical learning will occur. Ideally, faculty develop a specific curriculum-wide plan for how TPCAs and FCLAs are incorporated into each clinical course. In a concept-based curriculum the clinical learning focuses on the application of the concept or concepts in a specific clinical context; concepts are further incorporated into written assignments, discussions with the faculty member, and in clinical conference.

Creating a Lesson Plan

Developing a lesson plan for clinical teaching is similar to the planning that underlies classroom-based teaching. Specific clinical assignments are incorporated into the course syllabus and course materials so students have a clear understanding of what is expected of them. This also leads to increased consistency and accountability among faculty, particularly when multiple sections of the same clinical course are taught by different faculty. In addition to curriculum outcomes and course objectives, factors used to plan each TPCA or FCLA include the level/experience of the student, the type of clinical site(s), and the course placement (cycle) within the curriculum. Learning outcomes, concept(s) (and related competency) under study, expected student activities, and deliverables completed throughout the clinical experience should also be considered as part of the lesson plan. Use of a standardized lesson plan template for clinical learning helps achieve consistency from a curricular standpoint. Elements to include in clinical lesson planning are shown in Box 7.1.

Another important consideration is that in a contemporary clinical education model, students within a clinical group may be involved in different learning activities in different locations and on

BOX 7.1 ■ Elements of a Clinical Lesson Plan

- Activity name
- Targeted learning domain(s)
- Learning outcomes
- Concept(s) under study
- Clinical setting
- Activities to complete
- Role of faculty to facilitate learning
- Method of evaluation (written assignment, presentation, etc.)

the same or other days. In other words, some students may be doing TPCAs and other students may be doing FCLAs. Depending on the complexity, a FCLA may be completed by an individual student or within student teams. This approach allows for greater efficiency in the use of clinical sites with limited capacity.

Assignments

Assignments are an essential element of the clinical lesson plan. The purpose of an assignment is to promote the understanding of concepts and other information; promote thinking and clinical judgment; promote reflection on the experience, including an exploration of students' feelings, beliefs, or attitudes; and to provide a mechanism for feedback and evaluation. In a concept-based curriculum, concepts are purposefully planned as a component of the clinical assignment. There are many types of assignments that can be incorporated into TPCAs or FCLAs. Driving factors for determining the type of assignment include the clinical site, the type of learning activity, and the desired learning outcome. Common clinical assignments include a concept map, a concept analysis, case study, case presentation, nursing care plan, development of a teaching plan, reflective journal, short written assignments, guided worksheets, compare and contrast assignments, evidence-based practice assignments, and assessment assignments. A few of these assignments are discussed further below.

Concept Map. A concept map is a diagram of key concepts in the context of patient care or related to a situation and shows key relationships between the concepts. It allows students to explore the health conditions or factors affecting the patient and translate these into appropriate representative concepts and fosters the integration of multiple concepts into cognitive understanding; further, this strategy is credited with increasing student critical thinking and metacognition (Senita, 2008; Taylor & Littleton-Keamey, 2011). Concept maps can be used in the clinical setting as an individual assignment or as a collaborative assignment for both TPCAs or FCLAs. There are a number of ways concept map assignments can be created (Daley, Morgan & Black, 2016); thus faculty will need to develop parameters for such an assignment. Fig. 7.1 shows an example of a concept map assignment.

MISCONCEPTIONS AND CLARIFICATIONS

Misconception: All students within a clinical learning group should be involved in the same clinical learning activities on any given day to maintain consistency among the learners and to avoid confusing the nursing staff in the clinical areas.

Clarification: All students within a clinical group may complete the same clinical learning activities over the course of a semester or term, but students may be involved in different learning activities on the same day. Some students may be assigned to a TPCA, and at the same time other students may be assigned a FCLA.

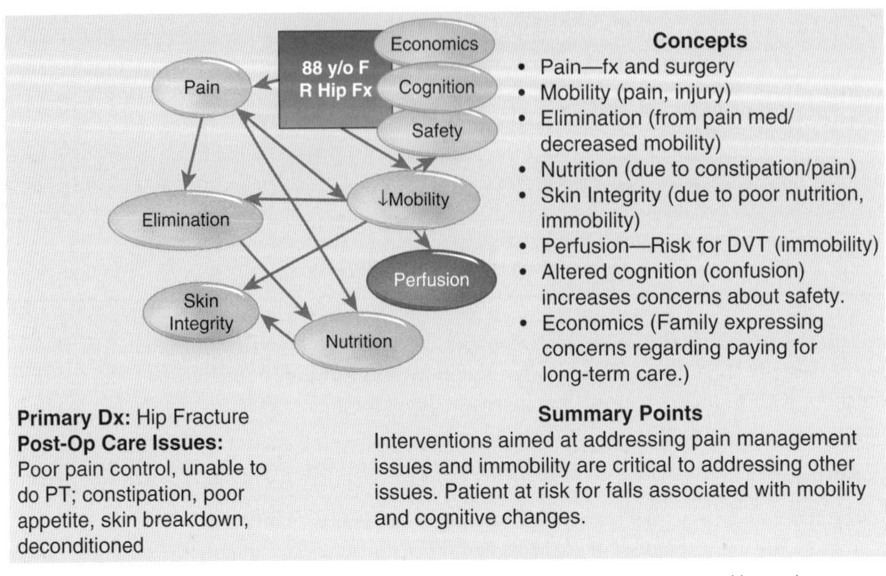

Fig. 7.1 The concept map is a common concept-based teaching strategy used in nursing.

Concept Analysis. Although a formal concept analysis involves an intense review and study of the literature, in an educational setting, students can do an analysis of a concept as it presents in a number of patients or situations to reinforce the commonalities of the concept.

Case Study and Case Presentation With Conceptual Focus. A case study is a written assignment with a focus on a single patient, family, setting, or situation. Students provide a written narrative of the events in the context of the major concepts involved following a template or assignment guide. In some cases, a concept map may be created to accompany the case study. A case presentation is similar but is more of an oral presentation—often done in a clinical seminar or during patient rounds.

Nursing Care Plan. A nursing care plan has been used for a number of years as an assignment in the clinical area. A typical care plan approach includes the identification of a nursing diagnosis, supporting data for that diagnosis, a goal, interventions to address the diagnosis, and evaluation. These elements are presented in a column format, with each diagnosis addressed independently in a linear format. Students prioritize three to five diagnoses for each care plan. The value of a care plan is that it helps the student learn the nursing process. Although care plans can still be used in a concept-based curriculum, critics suggest that a care plan limits thinking, approaches problems in a linear approach, and fails to address the reality of interrelated problems.

Teaching Plan. A teaching plan has been a common clinical assignment for years. In a concept-based curriculum, students apply relevant teaching and learning concepts to create a health teaching plan for a patient, family, or community. Although specifics of assignments may vary, a teaching plan typically includes a learner assessment, objectives, developing content, and consideration of appropriate teaching strategies for the target learner. These plans can be completed by students individually or as a collaborative assignment.

Reflective Journal. A reflective journal fosters reflective thinking, which is an underlying component for developing clinical judgement (Lasater & Nielsen, 2009b). This is typically an independent assignment where student think about the concepts involved in the context of the care they provided or the situation observed and then reflect on questions posed by the faculty member.

FACULTY ROLE/EXPECTATIONS

In most nursing programs, clinical courses are taught by both full-time faculty and part-time or adjunct faculty. One of the ongoing challenges is maintaining consistency and quality in the clinical learning experience. This is particularly a challenge for faculty unfamiliar with a concept-based curriculum. Transitioning instructors from a traditional approach to a conceptual approach, especially in the clinical area, represents a significant challenge (Giddens & Brady, 2007; Hendricks and Wangerin, 2017). Professional development of clinical faculty is encouraged; this is discussed further in Chapter 9. For excellent clinical instruction to occur, the instructor must have expertise in the clinical area he or she is assigned to teach, understand the conceptual approach, and follow the clinical course plan. Additionally, the instructor should be perceived as approachable (especially by the students), have excellent interpersonal skills, and possess clinical teaching skills. Two specific skills worth mentioning include guided thinking and assessing clinical performance.

Guiding Students to Think

One of the hallmarks of the conceptual approach is helping learners gain higher-order thinking skills. Clinical instructors foster higher-order thinking during clinical experiences by asking thought-provoking questions in a guided thinking process. Guided thinking can also be facilitated through well-designed clinical assignments.

Clinical instructors need to develop skill in questioning students to avoid making them feel as though they are being "grilled," leading to unnecessary stress. There is a tendency for faculty to ask low-level questions where the student merely repeats information they have gained (Phillips, Duke, Weerasuriya, 2017). Instead, faculty should encourage students to stretch their thinking beyond obvious answers. The use of open-ended questions that require students to explain their thinking, rationale, and linkage to concepts is desired. Guided instruction in clinical judgment is needed for students to learn to think like a nurse (Caputi, 2018; Konradi, 2012). Experienced nurses make decisions based on data. They know what information to collect, interpret the meaning of the data, and take appropriate action. When students enter a nursing program, they don't know how nurses solve clinical problems. They need guidance to learn what information is necessary to collect and how to use that information to make decisions that are situation and patient specific. Box 7.2 illustrates a clinical instructor guiding a student (who is involved in a TPCA) through active thinking and help them make cognitive connections to concepts in clinical practice.

BOX 7.2 ■ Exemplar of Guided Instruction for Clinical Judgment

Daniel, a junior nursing student, is completing a DPCA with a patient with the medical diagnosis of anemia. Daniel remembers that a patient with anemia has a decreased amount of hemoglobin, which results in decreased amounts of oxygen available to the body. He then thinks about the factual information regarding decreased oxygen and the attributes of the concepts of gas exchange and perfusion as well as to interrelated concepts. The nursing instructor asks Daniel, "What other concepts are affected by impaired gas exchange and perfusion for this patient?" He considers his options and replies, "Mobility, Nutrition, Anxiety, Fatigue, and Safety."

The clinical instructor encourages Daniel to confirm the presence of these interrelated concepts through further data collection and patient assessment. The instructor also encourages him to investigate the underlying cause of the anemia and other health conditions. Understanding the specific pathophysiology of the anemia and interrelated health conditions provides additional information for Daniel to consider for his patient.

Later, as a follow-up to the previous conversation, the instructor asks Daniel what additional concepts he has considered for his assigned patient. He mentions several other concepts including *Development, Culture, Functional Ability, Care Coordination,* and *Patient Teaching*.

As demonstrated with this example, Daniel reflects facts and other things he has previously learned to determine patterns. He considers information and analyzes this as part of clinical judgment. From a conceptual learning standpoint, this process facilitates cognitive connections, leading to deeper and transferable understandings.

Observation and Coaching

Students require feedback on an ongoing basis. Effective clinical instructors develop skill in accurately assessing performance and providing feedback and coaching in a constructive, nonthreatening way. Faculty should avoid premature conclusions based on first impressions; rather a series of observations is needed for an accurate assessment. It is particularly important that clinical instructors identify learning needs of students based on an accurate assessment and provide additional instruction where needed. End-of-course evaluation is also expected of clinical faculty. This is discussed further in Chapter 8.

Exemplars of Concept-Based Clinical Teaching Strategies

Conceptual learning in the clinical areas involves making purposeful connections to curricular concepts discussed in didactic courses. The large majority of concepts are evident in all clinical areas, so the only limits to learning are those placed by the faculty. Additionally, students will encounter clinical situations and patients representing important curricular concepts they have not yet formally learned about. This issue is no different than any other curriculum model. Faculty should plan to help students make connections to these concepts through other means. In all likelihood, the students probably have had some level of exposure or awareness to many things before having a formal concept presentation. For this reason, faculty should try to not overthink or be too prescriptive regarding conceptual learning in the clinical environment. Concepts are represented by a multitude of exemplars, so the goal is to help students learn from any situation. For example, if the students have studied the concept of *Gas Exchange* in the classroom, every patient encounter is an opportunity to deepen their understanding of *Gas Exchange*. Considering that *Gas Exchange* ranges from optimal to significant impartment of gas exchange and that the concept is evident in all humans across the life span and in every clinical setting, a learning activity in *Gas Exchange* does not require assigning a student to a patient in respiratory distress. Students can learn about *Gas Exchange* from patients who have optimal and impaired gas exchange.

As discussed earlier in this chapter, faculty should develop and prepare lesson plans for all areas of clinical learning. By doing so, greater consistency is gained and also a greater ability to track expected clinical learning outcomes. This section provides examples for a variety of clinical learning activities with a conceptual lens.

CONCEPT-FOCUSED ACTIVITIES

Safety

Safety is a core concept that should be purposefully incorporated into clinical learning. An example of a FCLA focused on the concept of *Safety* is presented in Box 7.3. Once completed, students should incorporate what they learned about safety on subsequent clinical days as part of the individual student's patient care experience. In other words, this is not a "one and done" experience—rather, this type of thinking should be continuously applied to learn the nuances and salient features within each patient context and within each type of health care environment. Over time *Safety* becomes a foundation of practice.

Mobility

Box 7.4 is an example of a FCLA associated with the concept of *Mobility* with a compare-and-contrast focus. During this activity students analyze data and assess three patients to determine whether their level of mobility is expected and acceptable, as well as identify risks. By collecting

BOX 7.3 ■ FCLA for the Concept of Safety

National Patient Safety Goals in the Clinical Setting

Lesson Objective: Assess how the National Patient Safety Goals are applied in the clinical setting.

Amount of time for learning activity: 4 hours.

Clinical Preparation: Locate and download the current *National Patient Safety Goals* from The Joint Commission website. Review the goals (simplified version) in each of the areas (ambulatory care, behavioral health care, etc.) and notice commonalities across clinical sites. Bring a copy of the goals that most closely link with the clinical site you will be in.

Activity to complete: Review the National Safety Goals and find evidence that actions are being taken within the clinical site to meet the goals and protocol. Specifically, address the following questions.

- For each goal, describe the actions you observed nurses and other health care providers take to meet the goal. Also note if you saw inconsistency in practice.
- Were there any goals you were unable to assess? If so, which ones? For goals you were unable to directly assess, discuss with nurses in the care environment how they would ensure achievement of those goals. Compare their answers to national safety guidelines.
- What factors regarding the environment indicate that these safety goals are being met?
- What factors regarding the environment indicate a need for change so the safety goals can be met?
- Complete and submit the worksheet for this assignment located in your course materials and address the questions listed above. Be prepared to share your experiences with the clinical group during debriefing in post-conference.

Adapted from: Caputi (2018). Think Like a Nurse: a Handbook. Rolling Meadows, IL, Windy City Publishers.

BOX 7.4 ■ FCLA for the Concept of Mobility

Evaluating Patient Activity Level

Concepts: Mobility, Clinical Judgment

Lesson objective: Compare and contrast the activity level of three patients to determine acceptable ranges and identify appropriate nursing interventions.

Related competency: Develop clinical judgment to ensure accurate and safe care.

Activity to complete:

- Collect the following data that may affect activity level of three assigned patients: age, gender, health conditions that brought the patient to the health care setting, information about the health condition that may influence activity level, other pre-existing conditions and their effect on the activity level, medications the patient is currently taking, information about the medications that may affect activity level, level of pain the patient may be experiencing, procedures the patient experienced while in the health care setting and the effect of those procedures on activity level. Also, determine whether there is a specific notation in the physician orders, physician notes, or nurses' notes regarding the patient's activity level. If possible, determine what the level of activity has been for each patient during the past 24 hours. If the patient is ambulatory, assess the patient's gait, balance, posture, and ease of movement.
- During post-conference, briefly present the first patient in a case format. After presenting all the information, discuss the patient using the following guiding questions: a) Is the level of activity acceptable? Why? Why not? b) What level of activity can be expected for the patient without causing harm? c) If the patient is not able to engage in the expected level of activity or if the patient's level of activity potentially could lead to harm, what actions should be taken? What consequences could occur? Present the second patient and third patients using the same approach. Compare the first, second, and third patients with a discussion about why the activity level for each patient may vary.
- Complete and submit the worksheet for this assignment located in your course materials and address the questions listed above.

BOX 7.5 ■ FCLA for the Concept of Perfusion

Concept: Perfusion

Lesson objective: Compare and contrast perfusion as it presents in three patients.

Related competency: Retrieves appropriate information from the health record; conducting a health assessment; clinical judgement

Activity to complete:

Complete an in-depth analysis of perfusion on three assigned patients. Your activities should include a review of a health record (if available), patient assessment, and review of care. Complete the following table to organize your thoughts. How are the patients similar and different with regard to perfusion?

	Patient 1	Patient 2	Patient 3
Gender, Age			
Existing Health Conditions			
Information from health record related to Perfusion			
Health Assessment Data related to Perfusion			
Interventions to support perfusion			
Conclusion: optimal, impaired, or at risk for impaired perfusion?			

the appropriate data and then making interpretations and inferences about the data, students arrive at conclusions that guide actions in clinical practice. This analysis, interpretation, and decision-making help to facilitate clinical judgment.

Perfusion

Perfusion is a concept that can be applied to any patient in any setting—because, students can learn about perfusion from people who have optimal perfusion, as well as impaired perfusion. Box 7.5 is an example of a FCLA for the concept of perfusion that is intended to deepen students' recognition of how perfusion presents in the clinical setting in a variety of patients. Specifically, students assess individuals to determine whether they have optimal or impaired perfusion and assess risk factors for impaired perfusion. They also evaluate the care to determine which interventions (if any) support perfusion and the effectiveness of those interventions.

Health Care Systems

A number of concepts link to health care systems such as *Health Care Organizations, Health Care Economics, Health Policy, Ethics, Safety, Health Care Quality,* and *Technology and Informatics.* The traditional model for clinical instruction places the students in patient' rooms for the majority of the time they are in the clinical setting, and thus their learning tends to be limited to the perspective of the individual nurse and perhaps the unit of care. Students have often missed opportunities to learn about these concepts on a systems level. Spector and Echternacht (2011) report that a number of studies have cited actual errors and near misses that have resulted from a lack of familiarity with the workplace environment. Box 7.6 provides an example of a FCLA focusing on the concepts of *Health Care Quality and Safety*. In this example, the students review the concept in the context of medication administration from the perspective of the individual nurse, the unit of care, and at the system level. The importance of safe administration of medications cannot be overemphasized. However, because of time constraints, many faculty focus exclusively on the actual psychomotor skill of administering medications. Although psychomotor skills are important, students completing a

BOX 7.6 ■ FCLA for Medication Administration Safety

Administration of Medications from a Unit and Systems Perspective.

Concepts: Safety, Health Care Quality

Lesson Objective: Analyze the clinical area to learn about best practices in medication delivery process and determine possible sources of medication errors.

Amount of time for learning activity: 4 hours

Activities to complete:

1. For the first 3 hours, follow a nurse and specifically observe him/her in regard to the administration of medications. Watch and note every step of the process, including the process for new medication orders, the processing of the medication order into the system, reviewing the order, retrieving the medication, administration of the medication, documentation, and observing for evidence of the effects. Be sure to also notice how the nurse manages multiple patients, resources used for safe medication delivery, and the system used to keep track of time for medication delivery.
2. As appropriate, ask clarifying questions to learn as much as you can regarding the process. Also discuss with the nurse the most common medication errors made on that unit and biggest challenges associated with medication management. Also talk with a pharmacist to gain an alternative perspective.
3. During the last hour, create an illustration or flow chart to represent medication administration process, incorporating system factors and unit of care factors.
4. Be prepared to share your experiences with the clinical group during debriefing in post-conference. Be sure to describe things observed to ensure safe medication delivery. Also discuss areas where potential errors could occur and things that could be done to reduce the possibility of error.
5. Write a 2-page reflection paper on your experience including things you observed such as roles of various team members, evidence of adherence to medication administration protocol, areas where errors could have occurred, what you learned from the experience, and how you will incorporate what you learned into your practice moving forward. Submit your flow chart with your paper.

learning activity such as this gives students great insight regarding the entire process of medication administration. Students learn ways to not only to avoid errors in medication administration but to identify potential problems and work to resolve them before an error is made.

Other Concept-Focused Activities

Concept-focused learning activities can be developed for any of the nursing concepts in the clinical setting. Appendix A presents several additional examples of concept-focused learning activities including *Evidence, Patient Education, Health Care Organization, Health Care Quality, Technology and Informatics, Infection, Collaboration*, and *Culture*.

MISCONCEPTIONS AND CLARIFICATIONS

Misconception: Designing concept-based teaching strategies for the clinical environment is challenging because the concepts must be present in the clinical environment in a similar order as concepts are presented in the curriculum.

Clarification: A concept-based approach actually allows for much greater flexibility for learning compared to a traditional content-focused curriculum. Nearly all nursing concepts presented in a nursing curriculum are in all clinical sites every day! For this reason, matching concepts in the clinical area to the sequencing of concepts in the curriculum is not an issue. As students learn concepts in didactic courses, specific concept exemplars are presented in class. The clinical environment represents a multitude of other exemplars of the same concept to extend and deepen learning. In other words, the clinical environment allows students to see how that concept applies in other ways.

Other Concept-Based Teaching Strategies for the Clinical Settings

PATIENT ASSESSMENT

Patient assessment is usually introduced in the nursing skills laboratory and students continue to learn and develop their skills in patient care areas. As discussed in Chapter 6, a nurse's approach to patient assessment involves thinking conceptually. To help move students from a task-oriented approach of assessment to thinking like a nurse, students require deliberate guidance. Table 7.2 provides an example of a TPCA focused on patient assessment and the recognition/identification of priority concepts. The patient data sheet organizes the assessment data conceptually. Note how this patient data sheet relates back to the thinking flowchart presented in Box 6.1 in Chapter 6. This arrangement of patient data represents the nurse's thinking and requires a deep understanding of concepts to determine individual patient needs.

An alternative approach is to ask students to conduct an assessment of a patient and identify patient needs without any prior knowledge of the patient or the patient's condition. Students are assigned a patient upon entering the clinical areas. Prior to receiving report, the student conducts an assessment on an assigned patient. At the completion of the assessment the student lists everything observed and considers which concepts of concern are represented by the assessment data; the student also identifies interrelated concepts for each of the identified concepts. From the list of concepts, nursing actions (such as gather more data from laboratory reports or review the medication administration record) and nursing interventions to address the identified concepts are determined and prioritized. After completing the assessment, the student receives a report from the nurse and then completes direct patient care. This activity encourages the student to independently identify issues, problems and then gain clarification regarding those issues based on the report. This activity helps students practice "seeing beyond the report."

Table 7.2 ■ **Example of a DPCA for Patient Assessment.**

Conduct an assessment on your assigned patient. After completing the assessment, document your findings in the patient health record. Next, complete the table below, related to priority concepts identified as part of the assessment

Concepts of Concern	**Areas of Concern R/T the Concept**	**What other information should you collect r/t this concept?**	**What interrelated concepts are present?**	**What interventions should you carry out for *this patient* r/t this concept of concern?**	**What should you report about this concept issue and to whom?**

Thinking Skills: What thinking skills and strategies did you use when completing this assignment? Explain.

CLINICAL NURSING SKILLS

In a traditional curriculum, clinical nursing skills are often taught initially in a nursing skills laboratory setting as one of the early courses in the curriculum. In a concept-based curriculum, nursing skills may still be taught in an early nursing course, or they may be integrated into courses throughout the nursing program and taught as part of a concept overview. Regardless, students should gain confidence performing the skill correctly and that they understand the context of the skill as a nursing intervention and how this factors into patient care through a conceptual lens. For this reason, faculty should be intentional about planning opportunities for students to discover linkages between nursing skills and concepts. Students continue to practice skills in the patient care areas under the supervision of the clinical faculty and may be linked to expected clinical competencies. Box 7.7 presents an example of a learning activity that can be done in a patient care area or in a simulation lab as a way to help nursing students think though nursing skills and linkages to appropriate concepts.

INTEGRATED LEARNING THROUGH TOTAL PATIENT CARE

As mentioned previously, there is still a need for students to have learning experiences providing total patient care. The process of providing total patient care involves the integration of multiple concepts. Students generally are assigned one or more students and complete the care of the patient(s) over the course of a shift or a part of a shift. The two most common written assignments associated with total patient care are a care plan and concept map. A care plan is a process whereby the students assess the patient to identify nursing diagnoses, set care goals, determine appropriate interventions and then evaluate the interventions. Although these are still common assignments, the usefulness for stimulating higher-level thinking has come into question (Oermann Shellenbarger & Gaberson, 2018). In a concept-based curriculum, a concept map is a common a written clinical assignment for students involved in total patient care. An example of a concept map written assignment is shown in Figure 7.1. There are a number of templates used for concept maps; these are discussed further in Chapter 6.

BOX 7.7 ■ Enhance Clinical Judgment Related to Nursing Skills

A student is assigned to assess multiple patients chosen by faculty to determine how to safely alter selected nursing skills procedures learned in the skills laboratory. (It is best if the patients selected are being cared for by other students in the clinical group to promote engaged discussions during post-conference). The faculty selects two or more nursing interventions that have been ordered for the patient (for example, starting an intravenous infusion, inserting a Foley catheter, giving an oral medication, etc.), and then the students engage in the following activities:

1. Review the procedure for each selected intervention.
2. Assess each of the assigned patients and determines how each of the should be completed. The students should also determine what modifications if any would be needed based on each individual patient situation using assessment data collected. For example, if the identified intervention is insertion of a Foley catheter and the patient is unable to assume a supine position, the student would discuss how the modifications needed to safely complete the intervention.
3. The interventions (and potential modifications) should be explained in terms of concepts.
4. Interrelated concepts for each identified concept of concern are identified. The student must explain how each interrelated concept is affected and addressed.
5. The complete activity is discussed in post-conference to enhance learning for all students.

BOX 7.8 ■ Sample Questions for Simulation Debriefing

Debriefing after a High-fidelity Simulation Experience

- What were the primary concepts of concern in this patient situation.
- What were the assessment findings that you considered highest priority? How did this affect your decisions and the priority for the nursing actions you completed.?
- Did the patient respond as you expected? If not, what surprised you? Why do you believe the patient responded in that manner?
- What did you do well? Reflecting on this experience, what could you have done differently to be more effective in the patient care? In what areas do you think you need further practice?
- What other concepts are often present in a clinical situation such as this?

TEACHING CONCEPTUALLY IN THE SIMULATION LEARNING ENVIRONMENT

A nursing program that has adopted a concept-based curriculum incorporates conceptual teaching in all learning environments, including simulation laboratories. The purpose of simulation is to provide meaningful learning experiences that are as close as possible to a real-world experience with debriefing and guided reflection on the experience. Simulation experiences can range from low- to high-fidelity. The term "fidelity" means how closely something resembles reality. Low-fidelity means the experience is somewhat close to reproducing what is real; high-fidelity means the experience is very close to reproducing what is real. Nursing programs use a combination of low- and high-fidelity simulation experiences as part of clinical education.

Conceptual teaching approaches within simulation can be accomplished by developing scenarios with an emphasis on a concept, or by creating complex scenarios involving multiple concepts. As an example, if there is a desire that all students have a simulation experience caring for a patient with impaired perfusion, simulation scenarios can be developed to feature a desired exemplar of impaired perfusion (such as myocardial infarction or heart failure). If time allows, a series of simulation activities featuring different exemplars of the same concept could be completed, allowing students to experience variations in the concept, not only in the type of health condition, but also the age of patient, or the patient care setting. For advanced students, simulation experiences featuring *concept clusters* (meaning a group of interrelated concepts that commonly occur in clinical situations) provide the opportunity for students to gain experience managing patients with multiple needs and determining priorities. Simulations featuring concept clusters also represents another way to provide integrated learning experiences and assess learning outcomes.

A second opportunity to incorporate conceptual learning in a simulation is during debriefing. Because simulation provides students with clinical experiences that are close to a real-world experience, the same type of thinking that is taught and used in the patient care clinical setting should be incorporated in simulation. The tools presented in this chapter for use in the clinical setting can be adapted to high-fidelity simulation experiences. Guidance during debriefing should focus the thinking process for clinical decision making as it relates to the concept. Box 7.8 provides examples of elements related to conceptual thinking that can be used as a guide during simulation debriefing.

TEACHING CONCEPTUALLY IN COMMUNITY-BASED SETTINGS

As noted previously, concept-based learning should occur in all types of clinical settings. Faculty should develop TPCAs and FCLAs for students to complete in community, home health, and public health settings. In these settings, students apply the same concepts but the application context is different. Referring back to Box 4.4, *Health and Illness Concepts* are learned on the age continuum, the health-illness continuum, and the environment of care continuum, which includes community settings. *Professional Nursing Concepts* are learned from the individual nurse, the unit of care and, the system perspective. Likewise, the *Healthcare Recipient Concepts* are learned from the perspective of the individual, family, and community. The community learning experiences are the only way for students to truly learn the full scope of concepts in each of these categories. A simple FCLA in a community setting would be for students to review one or more concepts previously learned and consider the concepts in the context of community-based care. The student determines how each assigned concept applies to the community as patient or caring for patients within the community. As an example, a FCLA for a home health setting could be developed requiring students to compare the safety checks used in a home setting to those performed in an outpatient setting and an inpatient setting.

INTERPROFESSIONAL EDUCATION (IPE)

Nurses represent the largest group of health care professionals involved in the delivery of health care. Effective delivery of comprehensive, quality and efficient health care depends on high-functioning health care teams. The hallmarks of effective health care teams are reflected in the competencies proposed by the Interprofessional Education Collaborative (IPEC) and include interprofessional teamwork and team-based practice, interprofessional communication practices, and values and ethics for interprofessional practice (which includes an awareness and appreciation for unique roles, responsibilities, and contributions made by all members of the health care team) (IPEC, 2016). Nursing education must prepare nursing students to work within interprofessional health care teams. Because interprofessional teamwork is learned in the practice setting (Durkin & Feinn, 2017), intentional IPE learning experiences should be designed and incorporated in the clinical education curriculum based on the IPEC core competencies.

The IPEC competencies link to several professional nursing and health care concepts (*Collaboration, Teamwork, Communication, Ethics, Care Coordination*), thus there is great opportunity for IPE to be gained through clinical learning activities featuring these concepts. These should not be approached as an "add-on" to the curriculum, but rather incorporated as clinical teaching strategies (Oermann, Shellenbarger & Gaberson, 2018). Thus there should not be an expectation that all students have identical IPE experiences. Ideally students will share their experiences and reflections in a post-clinical conference. Specific learning activities can include simulation experiences (described previously) with other students from health care disciplines, observation experiences clinical rounding, and patient planning meetings.

Experiences in Areas of Exemplary Interprofessional Practice

Students can gain very robust IPE experiences through experiences in clinical sites where strong interprofessional practice (IPP) exists. Nursing faculty will first identify exemplary clinical sites where IPP occurs for optimal student learning. Areas where strong teamwork is typically seen include perioperative and surgery, rehabilitation hospitals and clinics, and mental health services. Many other clinical sites, particularly in community settings addressing health care access for underserved, or those addressing the health care needs of individuals with complex multi-morbid conditions also tend to have strong IPP. Box 7.9 provides an example of a FCLA using observation experience for IPE.

Patient Rounding or Patient Care Conferencing

Another learning activity to address IPE includes interprofessional patient rounding. This type of experience involves multiple health care professionals (such as physicians, nurses, pharmacists, dieticians, social workers, case managers) discussing each patient assigned to the team and

BOX 7.9 ■ FCLA for Interprofessional Education Activity

Observational Experience of Interprofessional Practice

Concepts: Collaboration, Communication, Care Coordination

Lesson Objective: Observe the members of the health care team for evidence of efficient interprofessional practice.

Activity to complete:

Spend the assigned clinical time observing all aspects of the clinical environment with an emphasis on the interactions and teamwork of the various members of the health care team. Specifically observe the following:

- The health care setting including the type of care provided and types of patients seen
- The health care professionals represented
- The roles and expertise of each member of the health care team
- Contributions of each team member in the delivery of care
- Patterns of communication between team members
- Examples of effective teamwork
- Challenges experienced and how the team worked together for solutions

As appropriate, ask clarifying questions to learn as much as you can regarding the clinical area and how the various team members work together.

After your observational experience, write a 2-page reflection paper addressing the things you were specifically asked to observe. Additionally, describe your impressions of the benefits and challenges working within the health care team and the level of respect observed among various health team members and the impact on health care outcomes.

working together to develop a plan of care. Although true rounding is most commonly seen in inpatient areas, interprofessional rounding may also occur in a modified format (such as a team conference) in other settings. Nursing faculty must gain the permission and cooperation from the clinical team leader conducting rounds (or unit where the patient rounds will occur) for the student to participate as a team member in the patient rounds. Students prepare for the experience by becoming familiar with the patients on whom rounds will occur. The students should be prepared to present and discuss the patients during rounding from a nursing perspective. Students should have an opportunity to share their experience in a post-clinical conference focusing on their impressions regarding how well the team collaborated, contributions made by various members of the team, and how members of the team collaborated in the decision-making process. Faculty should also consider asking the student to complete a written assignment based on the experience.

Summary

The clinical learning environment represents an epitome for students to apply concepts because this is where nursing practice takes place. Carefully planned learning activities within the clinical area provide the opportunity for students to expand their conceptual understandings. Concept-based teaching is implemented in all clinical settings using a variety of teaching strategies to engage students in meaningful conceptual learning. A combination of TPCAs and FCLAs that focus on one or more concepts in a patient care area should be developed and incorporated in all clinical courses. These activities must be deliberately planned to ensure students are engaged in learning that is focused on concepts as opposed to a focus on tasks and health conditions. A concept-based curriculum must focus on concepts in all learning environments, including the various clinical settings where nurses practice.

References

Caputi L. *Think Like a Nurse: A Handbook*. Rolling Meadows, IL: Windy City Publishers; 2018.

Daley BJ, Morgan S, Black SB. Concept maps in nursing education: a historical literature review and research directions. *J Nurs Educ*. 2016;55(11):631–639.

Durkin AE, Feinn RS. Traditional and accelerated baccalaureate nursing students' self efficacy for interprofessional learning. *Nurs Educ Perspect*. 2017;38(1):23–28.

Gaberson KB, Oermann M. *Clinical Teaching Strategies in Nursing*. New York, NY: Springer Publishing; 2007.

Giddens J, Brady D. Rescuing nursing education from content saturation: the case for a concept-based curriculum. *J Nurs Educ*. 2007;46(2):65–69.

Gubrud-Howe P, Schoessler M. From random access opportunity to a clinical education curriculum. *J Nurs Educ*. 2008;47(1):3–4.

Hendricks SM, Wangerin V. Concept-based curriculum: changing attitudes and overcoming barriers. *Nurs Educ*. 2017;42(3):138–146.

Institute of Medicine. *Future of Nursing*. Washington, DC: The National Academies Press; 2010.

Interprofessional Education Collaborative: Core Competencies for Interprofessional Collaborative Practice: 2016 Update. Washington, DC: Interprofessional Education Collaborative; 2016.

Ironside P, McNelis A. *Clinical Education in Prelicensure Nursing Programs: Results from an NLN National Survey*. New York, NY: National League for Nursing; 2010.

Konradi DB. Learning to think like a professional nurse: a critical questions strategy. *J Nurs Educ*. 2012;51:359–360.

Jessee M. Pursing improvement in clinical reasoning: the integrated clinical education theory. *J Nurs Educ*. 2018;57(1):7–13.

LeFlore JL, Anderson M, Michael JL, Engle WD, Anderson J. Comparison of self-directed learning versus instructor-modeled learning during simulated clinical experience. *Simulation in Healthcare*. 2007;2:170–177.

McNelis AM, Ironside PM, Ebright PR, Dreifuerst KT, Zvonar SE, Conner SC. Learning nursing practice: a multisite, multimethod investigation of clinical education. *Journal of Nursing Regulation*. 2014;4(4):30–35.

Lasater K, Nielsen A. The influence of concept-based learning activities on students' clinical judgment development. *J Nurs Educ*. 2009a;48(8):441–446.

Lasater K, Nielsen A. Reflective journaling for clinical judgment development and evaluation. *J Nurs Educ*. 2009b;48(1):40–44.

Nielsen A. Education innovations: concept-based learning activities using the clinical judgment model as a foundation for clinical learning. *J Nurs Educ*. 2009;48:350–354.

Nielsen A. Concept-based learning in clinical experiences: bringing theory to clinical education for deep learning. *J Nurs Educ*. 2016;55(7):365–371.

Oermann M, Shellenbarger T, Gaberson K. *Clinical Teaching Strategies in Nursing*. 5th ed. New York, NY: Springer Publishing Company; 2018.

Phillips NM, Dike MM, Weerasuriya R. Questioning skills of clinical facilitators supporting undergraduate nursing students. *J Clin Nurs*. 2017;26(23-24):4344–4352.

Senita J. The use of concept maps to evaluate critical thinking in the clinical setting. *Teaching and Learning in Nursing*. 2008;3(1):6–10.

Spector N, Echternacht M. A regulatory model for transitioning newly licensed nurses to practice. *Journal of Nursing Regulation*. 2011;1(2):18–25.

Tanner C. From mother duck to mother lode: clinical education for deep learning. *J Nurs Educ*. 2010;49(1):3–4.

Tanner C. Thinking like a nurse: a research-based model of clinical judgment in nursing. *J Nurs Educ*. 2006;45(6):204–211.

Taylor L, Littleton-Keamey M. Concept mapping: a distinctive educational approach to foster critical thinking. *Nur Educator*. 2011;36(2):84–88.

CHAPTER 8

Evaluation of Student Learning and Program Evaluation

Linda Caputi

Evaluation of student learning is a fundamental component of education. However, because learning occurs in the mind and thus cannot be directly measured or observed, student learning is difficult to measure. In the 1950s, a common behavioral theory definition of learning was that it results in a *change* in behavior and we can really only infer that learning has occurred on the basis of observed behavior. Although the idea of *change* is a common theme of most definitions of learning, the definition of learning has expanded since the early behavioral theory–based studies as a result of the influence of newer learning theories. Because this book focuses on the cognitive processing of students while they are involved in learning, a definition that includes the notion of change but also captures the higher-level cognitive processing by students is more useful. Oermann (2015) provides a definition of learning as "Learning is an enduring change in behavior, or in the capacity to behave in a given fashion, which results from practice or other forms of experience" (p. 16). Two critical components of learning are: 1) "learning is a process, not a product," and 2) "learning is not something done to students, but rather something students themselves do" (Ambrose, et al, 2010, p. 3). The definition and components align closely with the concept-based teaching strategies discussed in Chapters 6 and 7. The relationship between teaching and learning is that teaching is the arrangement of events so learning can occur. Therefore teaching involves the skillful sequencing of learning events for the purpose of students attaining the desired learning outcomes. The evaluation of learning is complex and requires a variety of assessment methods.

Evaluation of student learning is an important component of the conceptual approach, and this evaluation is performed at both the individual student level and the program level. Evaluation methods must ensure assessment of learning outcomes as they relate to the program's conceptual framework. This chapter expands on the information presented in Chapter 4 regarding program evaluation and presents best practices to evaluate student learning at both the course level and the program level to determine the effectiveness of a concept-based curriculum.

Program Evaluation Plan

As mentioned in Chapter 4, a program evaluation plan is designed as part of curriculum development and is a critical component in determining the effectiveness of a concept-based curriculum. The evaluation plan should be a proactive and systematic process that is used to determine the value or worth of the nursing program (Boland, 2015). Nursing faculty are familiar with curriculum evaluation plans as a key requirement for accreditation and state board of nursing requirements. These plans—which include assessment of curricular outcomes, frequency of assessments for which data are collected, analysis of the data, interpretation of the findings, and plans for using the data to guide program improvement (Accreditation Commission for Education in Nursing [ACEN], 2017a; Commission on Collegiate Nursing Education [CCNE], 2013; National

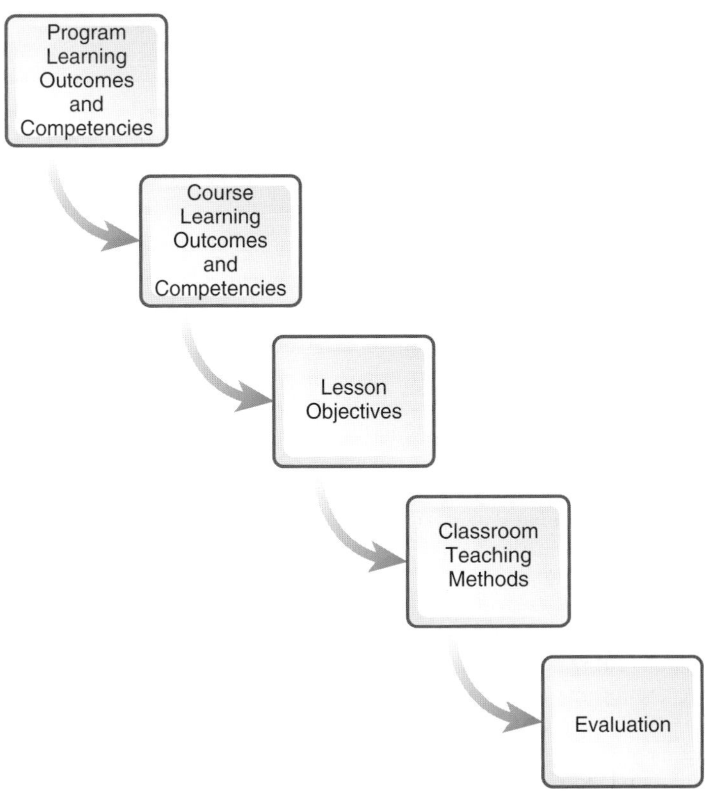

Fig. 8.1 Flow of learning outcomes from the program level to evaluation strategies.

League for Nursing Commission for Nursing Education Accreditation [CNEA], 2016)—can be applied to evaluating the effectiveness of a concept-based curriculum. If the data indicate that any of the outcomes are not being met, faculty should use these data to guide program changes. The two major areas of a program evaluation plan include assessing learning outcomes and program outcomes.

LEARNING OUTCOMES

Learning outcomes are "statements of expectations written in measurable terms that express what a student will know, do, or think at the end of a learning experience; characteristics of the student at the completion of a course or program. Learning outcomes are statements of learner-oriented expectations written in measurable terms that express the knowledge, skills, or behaviors that the students should be able to demonstrate" (ACEN, 2017b, p. 11). Learning outcomes flow through the curriculum and provide the structure for the evaluation of student learning (Fig. 8.1).

There are two overall types of learning outcomes: program learning outcomes and course learning outcomes. *Program learning outcomes* (also referred to as end-of-program student learning outcomes [ACEN, 2016]) reflect the characteristics or attributes of the students at the end of the nursing program. These learning outcomes represent the types of behaviors and activities students are able to engage in by the end of the curriculum. In the past, program learning outcomes were called "terminal objectives," an old term that is no longer used in nursing education with an outcomes-based curriculum. *Course learning outcomes* reflect the characteristics or attributes of the students at the end of a nursing course. Competencies may also be written for learning outcomes. Although learning outcomes are broad statements, competencies delineate the specific behaviors the student must achieve to demonstrate accomplishment of the learning outcome.

Program learning outcomes are carefully developed by faculty to reflect the nursing program mission, vision, and values (or philosophy), institutional educational expectations, and national standards related to nursing and health care. Once established, the program learning outcomes and competencies are used to develop the course learning outcomes and competencies. The course learning outcomes and competencies are then used to develop the course outlines and lesson objectives for each classroom session (Fig. 8.1). A course outline is developed that presents the concepts and exemplars, as well as teaching methods for each class session. The teaching session must engage the student in activities that require thinking at the cognitive level of the course learning outcomes and lesson objectives, and thus the course learning outcomes and lesson objectives must be written at the same cognitive level.

The final step illustrated in Fig. 8.1 is evaluation. Evaluation methods align with the expectations of the course. Many assessment methods are used to evaluate student achievement of lesson objectives that—because all curricular components are linked—are a measurement of course learning outcomes. Using a variety of methods to evaluate learning and program outcomes is not unique to a concept-based curriculum. The primary difference for the concept-based curriculum is that the evaluation methods must ensure assessment of learning outcomes as they relate to the program's organizational structure for content delivery, which is based on concepts. The assessment methods used to evaluate achievement of learning outcomes are varied and include examinations, clinical evaluation tools, formal papers, and student presentations as examples. The cognitive level of expected student performance measured with these assessment methods must align with the cognitive level of the learning outcomes. As students successfully complete each course in the nursing program, the course learning outcomes build to culminate in the program learning outcomes. Achievement of the program learning outcomes should then result in positive program outcomes, discussed in the next section.

PROGRAM OUTCOMES

In addition to learning outcomes, a program evaluation plan also addresses *program outcomes*. Program outcomes are "measurable indicators that reflect the extent to which the purposes of the nursing program are achieved and by which program effectiveness is documented" (ACEN, 2017b, p. 11). Measures used include graduation rates, time to graduation, NCLEX pass rates, certification examination pass rates, employer satisfaction and feedback on graduate performance, and graduate satisfaction and feedback regarding preparation for practice. If a nursing program curriculum is well planned and deliberately delivered, the program outcomes should be met through achievement of the program learning outcomes. A thorough discussion on program outcomes is presented later in this chapter.

MISCONCEPTIONS AND CLARIFICATIONS

Misconception: The conceptual approach requires completely different strategies to evaluate student learning.

Clarification: Faculty will continue to use many of the same evaluation strategies, but with a different focus. The focus of evaluation for the conceptual approach is the students' ability to transfer conceptual information from one situation to another. A focus on the application of an in-depth knowledge of concepts is at the heart of evaluation of student learning.

BOX 8.1 ■ Evaluation of *Collaboration* From Program Outcome to Class Evaluation

Program Learning Outcome
- Participate in collaboration and teamwork with members of the interprofessional team, the patient, and the patient's support persons.

Leadership Course Learning Outcome
- Compare and contrast techniques used to develop collaborative relationships with members of the interprofessional team, the patient, and the patient's support persons when caring for patients with complex, high-acuity conditions.

Class/Lesson Objective
- Analyze inter- and intraprofessional communication and collaboration skills used to deliver safe, evidence-based, patient-centered care.

Classroom Teaching Methods
- Concept presentation, Collaboration
- Case study review
- Small group discussion

Evaluation
- Classroom test items, in-class assignment, clinical evaluation tool

Evaluating Student Learning

It is the responsibility of the nursing faculty to determine if students have achieved the program learning outcomes by measuring achievement of course learning outcomes throughout the program using valid and reliable evaluation methods. The key to measuring student learning outcomes is that each evaluation tool should demonstrate a connection to a course learning outcome that relates to the concept-based curriculum. Student performance should be clearly linked to the application of the concept used in the curriculum. An example showing all elements from program learning outcomes through evaluation for the concept of *Collaboration* is shown in Box 8.1.

A central aspect of evaluating student learning in any curriculum, but especially in the concept-based curriculum, is the students' ability to transfer learning about a concept from one situation to another. *Can the students use what they have learned in a new situation?* Just as a child who learns multiplication tables must be able to determine when to use that math skill, so it is with the learning of concepts. Students who learn about a concept must be able to discern when knowledge of that concept should be used in a particular context as appropriate for safe patient care (Benner, et al, 2010). Evaluation methods in a concept-based curriculum should provide opportunities for students to demonstrate they are able to apply their learning to new situations. The methods used to evaluate student achievement of learning outcomes should link to the concepts so the evaluation of conceptual learning is clearly delineated. Examples of four common assessment methods are presented below showing how these are used to assess conceptual learning.

CLASSROOM EXAMINATIONS

One method for evaluating student achievement of course learning outcomes is a classroom examination. The faculty use a test blueprint that directly links a test item to the lesson objective, which is linked to the course learning outcome. If students are able to answer the test items linked to the lesson objective and the test items are determined to be reliable on the basis of item analysis, faculty can determine whether students are achieving the course learning outcome related to a given concept.

Classroom examinations cover concepts taught during the classroom sessions, as well as the exemplars used for concept application. For example, with regard to the *lesson objective* example in Box 8.1, a test item focused on the concept of *Collaboration* may have the following stem:

Present a patient situation. Then ask: Which collaborative action will the nurse take?

This question is focused on a patient situation while asking a question about the concept of *Collaboration*. An alternate approach to evaluating students' understanding of *Collaboration* is to present the question in the following way:

Present a patient situation. Then ask: Which action will the nurse take?

The actions listed in the options reflect a number of different alternatives, of which one represents a *collaborative* behavior without using the word "collaboration." This type of question evaluates the students' understanding of when to apply *Collaboration* to a situation.

The cognitive level of questions should match the course learning outcomes. The questions should assess the understanding of concepts via application and analysis of the concepts at a level appropriate to the course. For example, a simple application question may be:

Present a patient situation. Which concepts will the nurse further investigate?

The stem of this question does not ask about a specific concept; rather, students must draw from the patient situation the concepts that will be further investigated.

Questions directed at the application of concepts related to exemplars are also included on examinations. An example of a question related to the concept of *Pain* experienced by a patient during the postoperative period may be:

> The nurse assesses a patient 2 days after abdominal surgery. The patient reports diffuse abdominal discomfort. The nurse notes few bowel sounds, distention, and lack of flatus. *The nurse should implement which intervention?*

It is important to determine not only the concept but the cognitive level of the learning outcome and competency, then write the test item to match both. Table 8.1 provides an example of a test item focused on the concept of *Anxiety*. There are three versions of the test item, one written at the knowledge level, one at the comprehension level, and one at the application level, although all three focus on the same concept.

All the aforementioned questions represent a focus on concepts applied to patient situations. By using a test blueprint to link each question to a course learning outcome that represents specific concepts, the faculty can analyze test results to determine which questions were or were not effective at measuring student learning. This analysis should look at the individual student to provide individual remediation for the student. However, the analysis should also focus on how the students answered each question as a group. With this information, the faculty determines if remediation or reteaching of the concept is needed for the class as a whole (or considers the possibility that the test question was flawed). This analysis provides information about student achievement of specific learning outcomes and the concepts related to those learning outcomes. This information is necessary to guide the faculty's actions to improve the course on the basis of poor performance related to identified learning outcomes.

CLINICAL EVALUATION TOOLS

Clinical evaluation tools are commonly used to assess student performance. These tools are used to measure achievement of course learning outcomes as they relate to performance in the clinical environment. Again, if the course learning outcomes represent important nursing concepts, then evaluation of the course learning outcomes in turn evaluates student learning with regard to the application of the concepts used to build the curriculum.

TABLE 8.1 ■ **Example Test Item Focused on the Concept of *Anxiety* at Three Cognitive Levels**

Cognitive Level	Test Item
Knowledge (Remembering)	The nurse is caring for a 44-year-old patient admitted to the outpatient surgical center for a herniorrhaphy. Which assessment data indicates the patient may be experiencing anxiety? 1. Lab results indicate a fasting blood glucose of 96. 2. Heart rate 110; blood pressure 130/85 3. Respiratory rate of 12 4. Quiet tone of voice
Comprehension (Understanding)	The nurse is caring for a 44-year-old patient admitted to the outpatient surgical center for a herniorrhaphy. Which statement by the patient prompts the nurse to further investigate the presence of anxiety? 1. My girlfriend will be here soon and she would like to be with me when she arrives. 2. How many patients are having surgery today? 3. How long will I be here after the surgery? 4. My friend had this same surgery and ended up in the ICU.
Application (Applying)	The nurse is caring for a 44-year-old patient admitted for a herniorrhaphy. The patient's vitals are: BP: 140/90, P: 90, T: 98.4; R: 22. The patient tells the nurse this is his first experience with surgery. What is the nurse's first action? 1. Check the chart for the surgical consent. 2. Discuss postoperative care of the incision. 3. Assess the patient's ability to walk to the bathroom for a urine specimen. 4. Ask if he has specific concerns he would like to address at this time.

BOX 8.2 ■ **Focused Clinical Learning Activity: Concept Collaboration**

Collaboration and Conflict Resolution

- Interview a nurse and one other health care professional to describe an area of conflict in the clinical area they have experienced among other health care professionals and how the conflict was resolved.
- Observe the interactions of all the health care professionals on the unit. What conflicts did you observe? How were they handled or not handled?
- What conflict resolution principles were evident in the situations described to you by the nurse and health care professional and those you observed on the unit? How would you approach these conflicts? Explain your approach incorporating conflict resolution principles.

Continuing with the example of *Collaboration*, an item on the clinical evaluation tool is developed to evaluate this concept. The course learning outcome presented earlier can be used for this purpose: *Compare and contrast techniques used to develop collaborative relationships with members of the interprofessional team, the patient, and the patient's support persons when caring for patients with complex, high-acuity conditions.*

Students then engage in clinical activities that demonstrate their ability to analyze *Collaboration* among health care team members. Box 8.2 presents a focused clinical learning activity (FCLA) featuring collaboration that directs students to observe the activities and behaviors of the interprofessional team for the purpose of learning to deal with conflict, an important communication skill used when engaging in a collaborative relationship. The activity is best evaluated with a grading rubric (Table 8.2) that increases objectivity and consistency in the evaluation process.

TABLE 8.2 ■ **Grading Rubric for Conflict Resolution Clinical Activity**

Performance Criteria	Satisfactory: 2 Points	Needs Improvement: 1 Point	Unsatisfactory: 0 Point
Conflicts identified on the unit	Clearly describes conflicts on the unit	Descriptions of conflicts on the unit are vague and unclear.	Unable to describe any conflicts on the unit
Explanation of how to resolve a conflict	Clearly and accurately explains how to handle the conflict	Explanation of handling the conflict is scant and not well substantiated.	Unable to explain how to handle the conflict

BOX 8.3 ■ **Sample Paper Guidelines for the Concept of Collaboration**

Goal of Assignment: Compare and contrast *Collaboration* among members of the health care team in two health care settings.

1. Using the following three attributes of the concept of *Collaboration*, discuss how collaboration among the members of the health care team in each of the settings was similar and how it was different.
    - Roles and responsibilities
    - Communication
    - Teams and teamwork
2. For the concept of *Collaboration*, choose two interrelated concepts. Discuss how they were exemplified in each of the settings. Discuss how the settings were the same and different.
3. Draw conclusions about the collaboration you experienced in each of the health care settings. Discuss and explain why you would choose one setting over the other. Provide rationales for your selection.

The evaluation of a learning activity such as this can be used as a measure of individual student performance or evidence of learning for a group of students. To determine whether the class as a group is meeting expected outcomes on an assignment, an aggregate score is calculated among all students completing the assignment and evaluated against a predetermined metric. For example, if the predetermined metric is that 90% of the class achieves "satisfactory," then the aggregate mean score would be 1.8 or higher. Alternatively, the faculty can determine the total number of students achieving satisfactory divided by the total number of students in the class to determine whether the 90% metric is achieved. The aggregate score provides information about the level of learning for the class, indicating areas of strength and weakness of the assignment, the course, or the curriculum. Any indication of poor performance prompts faculty to determine changes that might be made to enhance the students' learning of the concept of *Collaboration*.

WRITTEN ASSIGNMENTS

Written assignments are a commonly used evaluation method. Formal papers provide opportunities for students to demonstrate not only their knowledge of a concept but their ability to apply higher-level thinking. Once again using the concept of *Collaboration*, a writing assignment is developed. The course learning outcome presented earlier can be used for this purpose:

> *Compare and contrast techniques used to develop collaborative relationships with members of the interprofessional team, the patient, and the patient's support persons when caring for patients with complex, high-acuity conditions.*

TABLE 8.3 ■ **A Sample Grading Rubric**

Grading Rubric	Excellent: 3 Points	Good: 2 points	Fair: 1 Point	Unacceptable: 0 Points
1. Using three attributes of the concept of *Collaboration*, discuss how collaboration among the members of the health care team in each of the settings was similar and how it was different.	Discussion is complete, explicit, and focused.	Discussion is complete and clearly written with minor areas incomplete.	Discussion is generally complete but lacks significant information.	Discussion is scant, superficial, and lacking in detail.
2. For the concept of *Collaboration*, choose two interrelated concepts, discuss how they were exemplified in each of the settings, and discuss how the settings were the same and different.	Discussion is complete, explicit, and focused.	Discussion is complete and clearly written with minor areas incomplete.	Discussion is generally complete but lacks significant information.	Discussion is scant, superficial, and lacking in detail.
3. Draw conclusions about the collaboration you experienced in each of the health care settings; discuss and explain why you would choose one setting over the other, providing rationales for your selection.	Discussion is complete, explicit, and focused.	Discussion is complete and clearly written with minor areas incomplete.	Discussion is generally complete but lacks significant information.	Discussion is scant, superficial, and lacking in detail.

The purpose of this written assignment (Box 8.3) is for the student to compare and contrast collaboration among the interprofessional team members in two health care settings. A grading rubric used to evaluate student performance on the assignment is presented in Table 8.3. An assignment like this would be appropriate for a course at the upper level because it requires students to have had clinical experiences in several different agencies or on several different units in one health care agency.

CONCEPT MAPS TO EVALUATE CONCEPTUAL LINKAGES

Concept maps are a helpful formative evaluation tool. A concept map is a visual tool that requires the student to organize information and make connections (Caputi & Blach, 2008). Students begin their clinical experience with a concept map template (a simple example is shown in Fig. 8.2) by placing specified information about the patient in the center of the map and priority concepts as determined by the student. As the student works through the day—performing assessments, making decisions, deciding on interventions, and engaging in the work of a nurse—the student adds to the concept map, including linkages between and among the concepts. Faculty provide feedback as the student adds to the map throughout the clinical experience. This tool provides faculty with a wealth of knowledge about the students' understanding of concepts and linkages among interrelated concepts. It also provides faculty with insights into how the student is thinking. Faculty can provide immediate feedback, thus helping students refine their thinking while they are engaging in patient care.

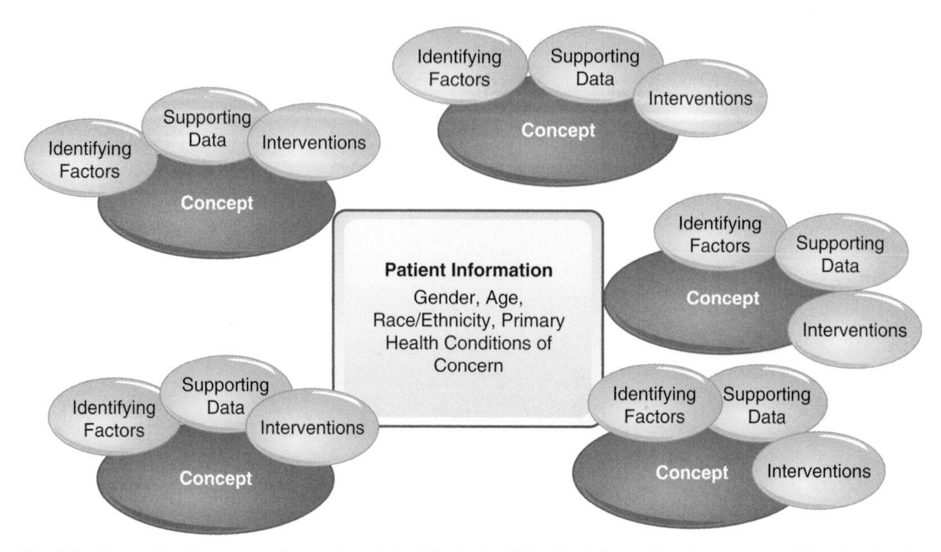

Fig. 8.2 Example of a concept map template. Students fill in the information (as requested by the faculty member) and draw arrows to show interrelationships among the concepts.

Program Evaluation

Program evaluation is a process that assesses program effectiveness through the assessment of program learning outcomes (which represent the types of behaviors and activities students are able to engage in by the end of the curriculum), as well as other standardized program metrics required by certification and regulatory bodies, earlier referred to as *program outcomes.*

MEASURING STUDENT PERCEPTION OF ACHIEVEMENT OF LEARNING OUTCOMES

Feedback from students about the effectiveness of courses in helping them achieve the course learning outcomes is imperative for ongoing program improvement. The completion of course evaluations by students is a well-established practice in education and should be used in the concept-based curriculum in addition to the previous evaluation measures discussed such as classroom examinations and clinical evaluation tools. Course evaluations completed by students are focused on the course learning outcomes. All course learning outcomes should be listed on the evaluation tool so students can rate how well they believe they achieved those learning outcomes. Other questions also can be included on the course evaluation, such as:

- Did faculty clearly make the connection between the course learning outcomes and the concepts that were taught?
- Did the teaching strategies engage you in activities to develop a thorough understanding of the concepts addressed in the course?
- Did the teaching strategies provide ample opportunity to apply concepts to nursing and patient situations in the classroom?
- Did the teaching strategies provide ample opportunity to apply concepts taught in the classroom to nursing and patient situations in the clinical setting?
- Did the evaluation methods used provide a clear understanding of your achievements based on the learning outcomes and further learning needs?

Other questions can be asked based on the needs of individual nursing programs. Of major importance is the students' evaluation of whether the course activities provided the opportunity to meet the course learning outcomes and learn the concepts presented in the course. It is imperative that all faculty use concept-based teaching strategies such as those described in this book. Students' evaluation of these teaching strategies is important because it answers two questions:

1. Were the teaching strategies effective from the students' viewpoint?
2. Did the students understand the purpose of the teaching strategies?

Students who value teaching strategies as important to their learning and understand the reasons for the teaching strategies used are more motivated to engage in the learning activities (Cannon & Boswell, 2016). This motivation is as important for clinical education as it is for classroom sessions. Both classroom and clinical experiences in the concept-based curriculum may be very different from students' previous experiences. Focused learning activities used in the clinical experience to enhance students' learning of a concept, such as the example provided for *Collaboration*, may not appear as important to students as spending time performing psychomotor skills. Therefore, it is imperative that faculty explain very clearly to students the importance of the activities to their learning.

MEASURING FACULTY PERCEPTION OF ACHIEVEMENT OF LEARNING OUTCOMES

Faculty evaluation of the curriculum is also an important component of the evaluation process (Giddens & Morton, 2010). The frequency of faculty evaluation of the curriculum depends on the evaluation plan established by the nursing program. Faculty complete a survey that asks questions about their involvement in the implementation of the program. It is important to solicit information about the success of teaching strategies, as well as problems encountered. Faculty are invited to provide suggestions based on data to improve the curriculum.

MEASURING PROGRAM OUTCOMES

As discussed at the beginning of this chapter, program outcomes are measurable, consumer-oriented indexes designed to evaluate the degree to which the program is achieving its mission and goals. A number of these measures exist. Some of the measures are easy to obtain and provide objective data, such as the first-time pass rate on the National Council Licensure Examination (NCLEX) and the completion rate. The employment rate is also an objective measure, but it is often difficult to obtain because of lack of contact with graduates. Equally important are data related to graduate and employer satisfaction. In this context, satisfaction refers to the belief of the graduate and employer that the curriculum was current and rigorous enough to educate nurses to provide safe, quality, evidence-based care.

NCLEX Pass Rate

Although the NCLEX pass rate for prelicensure nursing programs is reported quarterly in most states, the annual pass rate is used as the primary evaluation measure. All state Boards of Nursing and all three nursing accreditation bodies require a specific passing rate. However, the required pass rate varies among the state Boards of Nursing. Pass rate requirements are viewed as an indication of prelicensure program quality (Spurlock, 2013), and thus the NCLEX pass rate is a critical measure. All prelicensure nursing programs are responsible for providing students with a curriculum that prepares them for the NCLEX. A review of the detailed NCLEX test plan reveals the bulk of the test plan is based on concepts, and thus a concept-based curriculum is a practical way to prepare graduates.

When analyzing NCLEX pass rates, faculty should consider more than the annual pass rate to determine if the program is providing the education needed to earn a passing score on the examination. The National Council of State Boards of Nursing has a service available that provides each nursing program with a specific program report. These reports are important because they reflect actual performance on the NCLEX and provide a wealth of information about the scores of the school's graduates in specific areas of the curriculum compared with graduates from other programs. The specific areas align with many of the concepts in a concept-based curriculum. For example, the reports include the graduates' achievement in areas such as nutrition; elimination; comfort, rest, activity, and mobility; growth and development; and immunity, as well as many other areas that align with curricular concepts. NCLEX Program Reports are published twice a year allowing faculty to trend data over a number of reporting periods to identify areas that are consistently weak and for which curriculum changes should be considered.

Student Completion Rates

Nursing programs often use highly selective admission requirements resulting in the admission of students with higher qualifications than some of the other programs offered by the educational institution. Retaining students as they progress to graduation is a goal of nursing programs for many reasons. Nursing accreditation agencies consider completion rates as one key quality indicator. As one example, the CCNE guidelines require schools to have a 70% completion rate (CCNE, 2014).

Students should be able to complete the program within the time frame specified in the plan of study and successfully pass the NCLEX, so students can obtain employment and make use of their education as a practicing professional. Equally important and of primary interest to institutional and nursing accreditation bodies is the students' ability to repay school loans. For these reasons, schools have the responsibility to provide a curriculum that is achievable by students who meet the entrance requirements.

As faculty build a concept-based curriculum, they should plan classroom and clinical activities that are achievable. When developing classroom teaching strategies, faculty should expect students to engage in active preparation for class, which may include listening to narrated presentations, completing worksheets, and researching websites in addition to completing assigned readings. Faculty must consider the amount of time an average student needs to complete the class preparation assignments. A general guideline is that for each hour in the classroom, the student can be expected to spend 2 hours outside the classroom engaged in homework. Applying this guideline can help faculty plan assignments without overloading the student, which often leads to failure of the student to complete the work, thus jeopardizing his or her ability to complete the course requirements. A major advantage of the concept-based curriculum is the elimination of unnecessary content that leads to an oversaturated curriculum and student frustration (Giddens & Brady, 2007). These are major considerations that have an impact on the completion rate, which is an important program outcome measure.

Employment Rate and Employer Satisfaction

Another goal of a quality nursing program is a high rate of employment of the graduates. The employment rate is closely tied to the employer satisfaction rate. When employers are satisfied with graduates of a nursing program, they hire those graduates rather than graduates from programs with lower satisfaction rates. Information about employer satisfaction is often difficult to obtain. The nursing program's Advisory Committee should include representation from employers of the program's graduates. Important roles of the Advisory Committee are to engage in discussion about the performance of graduates and determine the number of graduates hired. Employers are encouraged to be honest and share their opinions of the graduates' performance.

The nursing program Advisory Committee is also a source for input and feedback about the concept-based curriculum. Members of the Advisory Committee are stakeholders in the program because they have an interest in the program's graduates as potential employees or as clinical students in their facilities. For this reason, it is important to share the structure and basis of the curriculum with these Committee members and request their input about the concepts studied in the program. It may be helpful to list the concepts taught in the program and ask members of the Committee to rate the importance of each concept in their place of employment. This information can be used when faculty review curricular concepts and how much time to spend on each concept.

Employer satisfaction is also gauged through a formal survey. The survey should ask the employer to rate the new graduate's performance with regard to the behaviors and characteristics that are indicative of the program learning outcomes. These ratings inform the faculty about how well the program learning outcomes are applied in practice. Employers should also be asked to note any job responsibilities the newly hired graduates are expected to perform frequently but that they were not prepared to perform. This type of questioning provides information about elements that may be missing in the program. It is important to compare the results of the employer surveys for the concept-based curriculum to the results from the previous curriculum. This comparison provides information about the usefulness and effectiveness of the concept based curriculum.

Graduate Satisfaction

Graduate satisfaction is an important indicator of a quality program. Typically a survey is sent to graduates between 6 to 9 months after graduation. Many of the same questions included on the employer satisfaction survey can be included on the graduate satisfaction survey but from the perspective of the graduate. That is, graduates should be asked how well they can perform the behaviors and characteristics that are indicative of the program learning outcomes and if they have encountered any job responsibilities they are expected to perform frequently that they were not prepared to perform. A difficulty with these surveys is obtaining a high return rate. However, without obtaining information from the employers and the graduates, it is difficult to determine if the concept-based curriculum is preparing graduates for actual practice, even if they passed the NCLEX. As is the case with the employer surveys, the feedback from graduates related to the concept-based curriculum should be compared to the feedback from graduates of the previous curriculum.

Summary

Curriculum evaluation is an important and expected process for all schools of nursing. In a concept-based curriculum, it is particularly important the evaluation methods include assessment of the way the program is being taught. That is, are all faculty engaged in teaching the concept-based curriculum using concept-based teaching strategies? Assessing the implementation of the program is critical to ensure the students are actually experiencing a concept-based curriculum.

Program evaluation is particularly important when a new curriculum is implemented (Giddens & Morton, 2010). When a new curriculum is implemented, the program outcome of NCLEX pass rates is always a concern. Therefore careful collection and analysis of evaluation data are critical to determine a cause and effect between the new curriculum and program outcomes.

References

Accreditation Commission for Education in Nursing. *Accreditation Manual: 2017 Standards and Criteria.* Atlanta, GA: Accreditation Commission for Education in Nursing; 2017a. Retrieved from http://www.acenursing.org/resources-acen-accreditation-manual/.

Accreditation Commission for Education in Nursing. *Accreditation Manual Glossary.* Atlanta, GA: Accreditation Commission for Education in Nursing; 2017b. Retrieved from http://www.acenursing.net/manuals/Glossary.pdf.

Ambrose SA, Bridges MW, DiPietro M, Lovett MC, Norman MK. *How Learning Works.* San Francisco, CA: Jossey-Bass; 2010.

Benner P, Sutphen M, Leonard V, Day L. *Educating Nurses: A Call for Radical Transformation*. Stanford, CA: Jossey-Bass; 2010.

Boland DL. Program evaluation. In: Oermann MH, ed. *Teaching in Nursing and Role of the Educator*. New York, NY: Springer; 2015:275–301.

Cannon S, Boswell C. *Evidence-Based Teaching in Nursing: A Foundation for Educators*. 2nd ed. Sudbury, MA: Jones & Bartlett; 2016.

Caputi L, Blach D. *Teaching Nursing Using Concept Maps*. Glen Ellyn, IL: DuPage Press; 2008.

Commission on Collegiate Nursing Education. *Standards for Accreditation of Baccalaureate and Graduate Nursing Programs*. Washington, DC: Commission on Collegiate Nursing Education; 2013. Retrieved from http://www.aacnnursing.org/Portals/42/CCNE/PDF/Standards-Amended-2013.pdf.

Giddens JF, Brady D. Rescuing nursing education from content saturation: a case for a concept-based curriculum. *J Nurs Educ*. 2007;46(2):65–69.

Giddens JF, Morton N. Report card: An evaluation of a concept-based curriculum. *Nurs Educ Perspect*. 2010;31(6):372–377.

National League for Nursing Commission for Nursing Education Accreditation. *Accreditation Standards for Nursing Education Programs*. Washington, DC: Author; 2016. Retrieved from http://www.nln.org/docs/default-source/accreditation-services/cnea-standards-final-february-201613f2bf5c-78366c709642ff00005f0421.pdf?sfvrsn=12.

Oermann MH. *Teaching in Nursing and Role of the Educator*. New York, NY: Springer; 2015.

Spurlock D. The promise and peril of high-stakes tests in nursing education. *Journal of Nursing Regulation*. 2013;4(1):4–8.

CHAPTER 9

Advancing the Conceptual Approach in Nursing Through Evidence, Professional Development, and Interprofessional Education

Jean Giddens

Throughout this book, the conceptual approach is presented to help nurse educators successfully implement a concept-based curriculum and concept-based teaching practices. Effective and sustained implementation requires a commitment from the faculty, individually and collectively, to continually develop expertise in this area. This chapter presents an overview of the nursing literature to date and areas for further inquiry, considerations for the professional development of nursing faculty with proposed competencies, and the future potential for the conceptual approach to be adopted across health-sciences education.

What Do We Know About Conceptual Approach From the Nursing Literature?

Although conceptual learning has been well represented in the education literature for decades, the same cannot be said for nursing. With a few exceptions, the conceptual approach has only been evident in the published nursing literature for about a decade. The primary areas of literature include articles that describe the conceptual approach movement, articles describing concept-based curriculum development and implementation, articles describing outcomes, and articles describing teaching strategies to facilitate conceptual learning.

THE CONCEPTUAL APPROACH MOVEMENT

The current conceptual approach movement in nursing began in the mid-2000s; thus some of the first articles that appear in the nursing literature describe this phenomenon. One of the earliest articles in the nursing literature proposed the conceptual approach as a way to address increasing concerns regarding excessive content in nursing curricula (Giddens & Brady, 2007). Specifically, the authors described how a concept-based curriculum and conceptual teaching differed from a traditional nursing curriculum and teaching practices and how this approach could lead to a reduction in curriculum content. Brandon and All (2010) presented a theoretical basis for the conceptual approach through the lens of constructivism learning theory and student-centered learning. The authors postulated that a constructivist approach using concepts and active teaching promotes critical thinking skills and builds confidence among students. More recently, several articles have appeared in publications targeting practicing registered nurses to inform their readers about trends in nursing education that affect the preparation of new nurses entering practice (Allen, 2013; Goodman 2014; Troussman, 2015).

CONCEPT-BASED CURRICULUM DEVELOPMENT AND IMPLEMENTATION

A large number of articles published to date in the nursing literature describe the concept-based curriculum. Not surprisingly, these articles focus predominantly on description of the curriculum design (Giddens, et al., 2008; Hollinshead & Stirling, 2014; Patterson, et al, 2016; Poopla, 2012) or the process of curriculum development and implementation (Brady, et al., 2008; Giddens, Wright, & Gray, 2012; Hendricks & Wangerin, 2017; Hollinshead & Stirling, 2014; McGrath, 2015; Patterson, Crager, Farmer, Epps, & Schuessler, 2016; Popoola, 2012). Two of the articles (Hollinshead & Stirling, 2014; Poopla, 2012) describe a specific curriculum framework or model as part of the curriculum design process, whereas another (Deane & Asselin, 2015) describes the change process for a faculty adopting concept-based teaching using Bridge's change model as framework. Common themes include challenges associated with faculty making the adjustment to a new approach, and addressing concerns regarding competing demands in curriculum development. Gaining full commitment among faculty to adopt concept-based teaching strategies is a common barrier to success (Giddens, 2016).

CONCEPT-BASED CURRICULUM OUTCOMES

In general, curriculum evaluation is a topic with limited visibility in the nursing literature. Even less is written on the process of evaluating a concept-based curriculum or published program metrics. Common metrics for curriculum and program evaluation include first-time NLCEX-RN pass rates, standardized test measurements, time to graduation, graduation rates, and satisfaction (student, employer, and/or alumni).

Five published articles reported on NCLEX pass rates as a curriculum outcome after the adoption of a concept-based curriculum; four of these reported no change to the NCLEX pass rates (Duncan & Schultz, 2015; Lewis, 2014; Murray, Laurent, & Gontarz, 2015; Patterson, Crager, Farmer, Epps, & Schuessler, 2016) Conversely, Giddens and Morton (2010) reported a drop in NCLEX pass rates with the first student cohort graduating from a concept-based curriculum. However, the authors also reported a number of confounding variables (including a change in admission requirements, move from a 9-month to 12-month academic calendar, expansion of enrollment, and initiation of distance learning at an off-site campus) that made it impossible to determine what role, if any, the initial drop of those passing was caused by the change to a concept-based curriculum. Standardized test measurements using Assessment Technologies Institute nursing education test scores and critical thinking assessment scores were used to evaluate the effect of conceptual learning in a concept-based curriculum compared with a traditional curriculum. The researchers found no statistically significant difference between the two groups but noted that the method of instruction may have moderated the effects of the concept-based curriculum (Fromer, 2017).

Time to graduation and graduation rates are other important curriculum outcomes. The concept-based curriculum did not affect on-time graduation rates (Duncan & Schulz, 2015; Murray, Laurent, & Gontarz, 2015 Lewis 2014), although two studies (Lewis, 2014; Murray, Larent, & Gontarz (2015) reported statistically significant improvements in program completion. Giddens and Morton (2010) reported a 97.5% graduation rate from the first three cohorts of graduates from a concept-based curriculum; however, there was no indication whether this was a change from the previous curriculum offered.

Program satisfaction commonly includes student and employer satisfaction. Several authors reported strong student satisfaction as measured in end of program surveys among those graduating from a concept-based curriculum, but these were not comparative measures (Grooder & Cantwell, 2017; McGrath, 2015; Patterson et al., 2016).Two studies reported no changes in student satisfaction as measured by end of program survey (Lewis, 2014; Murray, Laurent, & Gontarz, 2015), whereas Duncan and Schulz (2015) reported lower mean satisfaction scores among the first graduating cohorts from a concept-based curriculum. Less information was reported on feedback from employers. Patterson and colleagues (2016) and Giddens and Morton (2010) reported positive feedback from the nursing community regarding student and graduate performance in clinical settings while Lewis (2014) reported no changes in employer, or alumni satisfaction.

Several other elements of curriculum evaluation associated with a concept-based curriculum are reported in the literature. These include evaluating for "concept creep"(or in other words, additional concepts being added to the curriculum) using a PDSA cycle (Laverentz & Kumm, 2017), assessment of critical thinking (Duncan & Schulz, 2015; Patterson et al., 2016); higher order thinking (Getha-Eby, Beerty & Obrien, 2015), self-efficacy (Duncan & Schulz, 2015) students' perceived preparation to work in diverse clinical settings (Hensel, 2017), clinical competence among RN-BSN students in Taiwan (Lee-Hsieh, 2003; Kao, Kuo, & Tseng), and student perceptions related to quality of teaching/instruction among faculty in a concept-based curriculum (Grooder & Cantwell, 2017; McGrath, 2015).

MISCONCEPTIONS AND CLARIFICATIONS

Misconception: There is an abundance of literature and evidence supporting the conceptual approach in the nursing education literature.

Clarification: Although the conceptual approach is well represented in the education literature, the same cannot be said for the nursing literature. Most articles published in the nursing education literature have emerged over the last decade. There is a need for robust educational research evaluating outcomes associated with conceptual learning.

ARTICLES DESCRIBING CONCEPT-BASED TEACHING AND LEARNING

A third general group of published articles in the nursing literature associated with the conceptual approach describe models or specific teaching strategies related to concept-based teaching or learning. Concept-based teaching refers to a process where faculty design learning activities that guide students through the study of one or more concepts, including unique aspects of nursing care related to that concept. Teaching strategies have been designed for both the clinical or classroom settings. In the clinical setting, concept-based teaching strategies are designed to help learners make connections between the concept, the nursing care, and patient outcomes as opposed to a focus the tasks of care associated with the clinical experience. Concept-based learning in clinical settings for nursing education was first reported by Heims (1990), who reported improved learning outcomes when purposeful concept-based learning assignments were developed and applied in the clinical setting. Other articles describe the conceptual approach as a basis for linking clinical learning to the classroom (Nielsen, Noone, Voss & Mathews, 2013; Nielsen, 2016).

The clinical judgement model is described as a foundation for concept-based teaching in the clinical setting (Laasater & Nielsen 2009; Nielsen 2009). Specifically, students focused on a specific concept for the clinical day; learning activities included study guides, patient rounds, and faculty evaluation and feedback. Authors reported that this approach increased direct contact time for students and faculty, with the opportunity for faculty to role-model communication, and allowed students to focus on one idea at a time. Authors also noted improvement in critical thinking as a result of concept-based learning in the clinical setting (Laasater and Nielson, 2009). Hardin and Richardson (2012) describe a model of conceptual teaching in a concept-based curriculum. The core components of the model for effective conceptual teaching include addressing misconceptions, building enduring understandings, and developing metacognition. The authors also provide a description of five teaching methods proposed for effective conceptual teaching including misconception and preconception check, the discrepant event, concept maps, approximate analogies, and check your knowledge. Kantor (2010) describes the use of another model, the KBD approach (which stands for come to *know*, develop a way of *being*, and *develop* a plan of care) as a successful student-centered teaching and learning tool for linking clinical and classroom learning in a concept-based curriculum. Another article reported positive student feedback and a positive correlation of test scores after adopting a conceptual approach to a nursing pharmacology course (Lanz & Davis, 2017).

The concept map is perhaps the most commonly recognized concept-based teaching strategy in nursing. Introduced in the education discipline in the 1960s by James Novak, concept maps organize information and show the relationship between ideas. This approach involves the integration of multiple ideas and concepts into cognitive understanding to extend the understanding. In nursing, concept maps show the relationship of concepts in the context of patient care, allowing the student to make important connections and learn interrelationships (see Figure 7.1). A number of articles in the nursing literature feature concept mapping in the clinical and classroom setting (Harrison & Gibbons, 2013; Senita, 2008; Taylor & Littleton-Keamey, 2011); this strategy is credited with increasing student critical thinking and metacognition.

Higgins and Reid (2016) reported the development of concept analysis diagrams for each concept in the concept-based curriculum which then were used as a foundation for concept-based teaching in the classroom or clinical seminars. The diagrams show antecedents, attributes, consequences, interrelated concepts and shows how nursing care interfaces with the concept. Components of nursing care include assessment, analysis, intervention, and evaluation. Concept analysis diagrams differ from concept maps in that these are visual representation of the concept as opposed to a learning activity where students draw a map showing interrelationships among concepts, and usually in the context of a patient. Teaching strategies for specific concepts are the topics of several other nursing articles including concepts in a professional development course (Nelson-Brantley & Laverentz, 2014) transitional care (Mood, 2014), and social determinants of health (Decker et al., 2017).

SUMMARY OF CURRENT LITERATURE AND GAPS

Based on the surge of published nursing literature during the last decade, a clear movement of conceptual approach in nursing education is evident. The literature would also suggest that application of the conceptual approach is occurring primarily in undergraduate, prelicensure education. There are many variations in concept-based curricula; thus these are not "cookie cutter" curricula; however, there are common attributes to all, including clearly identified concepts and exemplars. It is the organization of the concepts and exemplars within and across courses that vary.

One of the greatest barriers to curriculum reform is fear of failure and negative program outcomes. Faculty may assume that if NCLEX pass rates and other metrics such as program completion and time to graduation are "good," then there is little need for curriculum reform. The literature published to date suggests that changing to a concept-based curriculum does not negatively affect traditional program outcomes of NCLEX-RN pass rate, graduation rate, time-to-graduation, or student satisfaction. Findings also suggest that conceptual teaching practices may lead to improved learning—although no longitudinal studies exist. These findings may be encouraging to faculty considering a change to the conceptual approach.

A variety of concept-based teaching strategies appear in the nursing literature—the most visible being concept maps. This area of literature should continue to evolve so the evidence expands and nurse educators have examples of best practices in concept-based teaching and learning. Traditional direct measures of program quality, teaching quality, and learning outcomes may not be sensitive to the true outcomes of the conceptual approach—in other words the influence of the conceptual approach in clinical judgment, in team-based care, and long-term patient outcomes. The next important step in scholarly work for the conceptual approach will be to tease out such differences if at all possible.

Developing Nursing Faculty Expertise in the Conceptual Approach

The conceptual approach is still in an early evolutionary stage in nursing. It takes time for a new method to be accepted, and even longer for widespread proficiency among faculty to create optimal curricula with extensive and consistent incorporation of this approach into didactic and clinical courses. Most faculty are aware of the conceptual approach, and many nursing programs have recently adopted or are in the process of adopting this approach. Although an individual program has little effect on the profession as a whole, the collective effect of many nursing programs adopting the conceptual approach over time will lead to a tipping point by which we will begin to fully realize the benefit within the nursing profession.

Developing expertise in concept-based teaching requires deep understanding of each of the interrelated elements of the conceptual approach—that is, concepts, exemplars, concept-based curriculum, concept-based teaching and conceptual learning. It is the integration of these components that leads to deeper conceptual understandings and mastery of concept-based teaching. These are not learned in a sequential or linear approach, nor can these be effectively learned in isolation. Gaining an understanding of the elements of the conceptual approach tend to occur together and over time.

How do faculty develop skills and expertise in the conceptual approach? First, faculty members must be willing to shift their perspectives about teaching and the instructor role. The conceptual teacher might be best described as a *learning coach* who creates a learning environment where the focus is more on ideas than content, where the students are guided through a learning process in a way that stimulates synergistic thinking and where the learners demonstrate critical reasoning and the ability to make generalizations. Many faculty have deeply rooted ways in which they view education and the learning process; the conceptual approach may challenge (or be in conflict with) their longstanding assumptions. Thus, being open-minded to learning, being open to the advice and suggestions of mentors, and being fully engaged and committed to ongoing professional development are needed to truly attain expertise. Let's face it; many faculty, particularly those who have been in nursing education for a number of years, pride themselves as expert teachers. Some may feel vulnerable with the adoption of a process they don't fully understand—thus a natural reaction is to reject the idea. An environment must be fostered where these feelings and perspectives are acknowledged, yet not allowed to derail efforts for curriculum and teaching reform.

MISCONCEPTIONS AND CLARIFICATIONS

Misconception: Most faculty successfully master the conceptual approach in a short period of time, especially if they attend a conference presentation or workshop.

Clarification: Achieving mastery in the conceptual approach takes time—even for experienced faculty. Gaining a general understanding of the conceptual approach must be followed by an ongoing commitment to implement and maintain the curriculum and dedicate themselves to apply conceptual teaching practices, seek feedback, and actively reflect on the process for self-improvement.

Professional development for faculty is the first step toward developing competence in the conceptual approach. The goals of professional development are to cultivate and increase an understanding of the conceptual approach, and to extend expertise in conceptual teaching and learning. Traditional approaches for faculty development include attending conferences or workshops on the conceptual approach. These approaches help to increase one's understanding and enthusiasm for change, but they are not often effective for successful and sustained change. Developing competence in the conceptual approach requires time, and thus it is not realistic to attend one presentation or workshop and "get it" (although it would certainly be convenient of this were the case). One learns to teach conceptually by doing it, learning from the experiences (both positive and negative), and then improving on those experiences. This is not a passive process! Proficiency is developed through the experience of applying principles associated with the conceptual approach, and purposeful and deliberate reflection. This is usually most effective in conjunction with other faculty and mentors who are also committed. Erickson & Lanning (2014) specifically suggest the establishment of professional learning communities as an effective method to support faculty. Such communities can be formed among interested faculty within your school and could also include colleagues from other schools or other disciplines. Professional learning communities provide many opportunities for faculty to share ideas and experiences, to provide/receive feedback, peer evaluation, and coaching, or to discuss journal articles or books. Furthermore, such groups can provide suggestions or ideas for creative learning strategies, development of lesson plans, and evaluation process.

Attaining competence and expertise in the conceptual approach is a developmental process whereby over time faculty progress from novice to expert. This process is truly a journey with an unspecified endpoint—meaning the developmental milestones are not specified at a fixed time or distance. Faculty on this journey will progress based on many variables, but perhaps the most important is being truly committed to the process. This requires openness to learning and dedicating the time and effort for a continuous process of learning, applying what has been learned, receiving feedback, and reflecting on the experience.

CONCEPTUAL APPROACH COMPETENCIES FOR NURSING FACULTY

It is one thing to be able to list the five elements of the conceptual approach (concepts, exemplars, concept-based curriculum, concept-based teaching, and conceptual learning) and another to fully understand each element, how these elements are interrelated, and truly understand how the conceptual approach differs from traditional nursing education. Competencies are behaviors that provide a framework for faculty development and evaluation. Conceptual approach competences for nursing faculty are presented in Box 9.1 and can provide guidance in professional development.

BOX 9.1 ■ Nursing Faculty Competencies for the Conceptual Approach

Competency 1: Understanding, Support, and Rationale

Attains a deep understanding of the conceptual approach.

- Articulates individual components of the conceptual approach clearly.
- Describes how the conceptual approach differs from traditional nursing education.
- Explains the rationale, benefits, and challenges of the conceptual approach as a model for nursing education.
- Analyzes findings from research in nursing and other disciplines that support the conceptual approach.
- Engages in self-reflection related to teaching and demonstrates a commitment to ongoing professional development in the conceptual approach.

Competency 2: Concepts and Exemplars

Effectively uses concepts and exemplars as components of the conceptual approach.

- Demonstrates a solid understanding of what concepts are, the common categories of concepts used in nursing education, and levels of concepts.
- Describes characteristics of ideal concepts to use for nursing education.
- Differentiates concepts from exemplars and effectively links exemplars to the concept to deepen learners' conceptual understanding.
- Appreciates the value of using concepts as a way to frame nursing knowledge.

Competency 3: Concept-Based Curriculum

Designs, implements, and evaluates a concept-based curriculum.

- Applies change theories/strategies within the curriculum revision process.
- Engages and informs community partners and key stakeholders in the curriculum development process.
- Uses literature, research, and best educational practices to design and implement the concept-based curriculum.
- Clearly explains the curriculum, including how concepts and exemplars are organized and used within and across semesters and courses (didactic, laboratory, clinical).
- Develops measurable program outcomes and evaluates program effectiveness.

Competency 4: Concept-Based Teaching

Designs and implements lesson plans that incorporate best practices of conceptual teaching.

- Develops lesson plans for classroom/didactic courses and clinical/laboratory courses.
- Concept units include a concept overview so that learners know what the concept is, understand the context of clinical practice, recognize the concept, and know what to do.
- Concepts are taught in a logical and consistent way, building on critical knowledge/facts and skills, and incorporating guiding questions to facilitate conceptual understanding.
- A variety of student-centered teaching strategies that are appropriate to learner needs and desired learning outcomes are incorporated into the concept-based teaching plans.
- Teaching strategies are intentionally designed to be interesting and challenging for student engagement and requires learners to extend previously held knowledge to new situations, applications, and contexts.
- Exemplars and interrelated concepts are deliberately incorporated for deeper understanding of the concept.

Competency 5: Conceptual Learning

Creates a learning environment that optimizes conceptual learning and achievement of learning outcomes.

- Demonstrates a solid understanding of the neuroscience of learning including physiologic variables that affect learning.
- Creates a learning environment and fosters a learning process that is safe, stimulating, and rewarding.
- Challenges learners to make cognitive connections from previous held knowledge/skills to concepts, leading to synergistic thinking and the formation of generalizations.
- Uses a variety of strategies to assess student learning and achievement of outcomes; learners demonstrate the ability to transfer information from once situation to another, can effectively solve problems, and demonstrate competence in performance assessments.

Beyond Nursing: The Conceptual Approach for Health Sciences Education

This book has been written primarily from the perspective of, and for the purposes of, adopting the conceptual approach in nursing education. However, the conceptual approach should be considered more broadly. Chapter 1 presented the background of the conceptual approach and traced its origins to the work of Helen Taba and the education discipline. Although unique concepts exist in each of the disciplines, concepts may also be applicable across multiple disciplines. This is particularly true among the health science professions.

In 2003, the Institute of Medicine (IOM) published *Health Professions Education: A Bridge to Quality* (IOM, 2003) which called for health sciences education reform. It was recommended that five core areas be included in the education of all health professionals: patient-centered care, working in interdisciplinary teams, evidence-based practice, quality improvement, and information technology. These core areas are reflected as concepts in most concept-based curricula. In 2011, the Interprofessional Education Collaborative (IPEC) created core competencies to guide curriculum development across the health professions which were reaffirmed and refined in 2016. The IPEC competencies include teamwork and team-based practice, communication, values and ethics, and roles/responsibilities (IPEC, 2016).

To expand on this, multiple concepts such *Diversity* and *Inclusion*, *Professionalism*, *Health Policy*, and *Health Disparities* are found throughout the health sciences literature. All health professionals must also have an understanding of biobehavioral concepts such as *Gas Exchange*, *Mood*, *Mobility*, *Perfusion*, *Cognition*, and *Infection* to name a few—the list could go on. What these concepts represent is the same but what truly differs is how each member of a health professional team interfaces with each other when the concept is represented in patient care. Put another way, there are variations in the roles and expectations of health care professionals—yet, all encounter the same set of concepts within their professional practice. This is not to say that the only difference between nurses and other health care professionals are the interventions, and in no way should this be interpreted as a diminishment of nursing as a unique discipline. Historically, nursing has had a significant role health care delivery and is clearly established as a practice discipline.

MISCONCEPTIONS AND CLARIFICATIONS

Misconception: The concepts in a nursing concept curriculum are generally unique to the nursing discipline.

Clarification: Most concepts found in a nursing concept-based curriculum are actually applicable to all health sciences disciplines and could be considered as a foundation for interprofessional education. That said, nursing students enrolled in a nursing program offering a concept-based curriculum gain an understanding and application of the concept through the lens of professional nursing practice.

The case could be made for conceptual approach to become the model for future health sciences education. It would be a natural way to support integrated interprofessional education experiences and concepts also support competencies. Over the past decade there have been substantial attempts to incorporate interprofessional education in health sciences education; these have produced mixed results. The challenge of layering such experiences into existing and divergent educational structures of each discipline has made it difficult to achieve significant impact as evidenced by the limited emergence of strong and efficient interprofessional practice models in health care. True interprofessional practice occurs when members of the health care team function in a way where all members are able to fully contribute to the care delivery using their unique knowledge and skills nested within the discipline they represent with the expectation of achieving optimal patient care outcomes. Although this occurs in some settings, it does not happen nearly enough. Most students today experience some degree of interprofessional education and may have an opportunity to be placed in a clinical setting where optimal interprofessional practice is evident but for the most part, these primarily remain as desired goals within the academic context. If the goal is truly to transform health care delivery through high-functioning teams engaged in interprofessional practice, then we must align health professions education for that reality.

Summary

Nursing is leading the way in the adoption of the conceptual approach and thus, nurse educators are well-positioned to lead education reform in health sciences education. There is a need for ongoing educational research associated with the conceptual approach in nursing education and other health sciences. Specifically, there is a need for the extension of best practices to support concept-based teaching and learning, and more evidence regarding outcomes for learners and programs. Through ongoing professional development, nurse educators should increase individual and collective expertise in the conceptual approach movement. Faculty have the ability to influence future generations of the nursing workforce equipped with higher-order thinking skills. With the evolution of concept-based interprofessional education, nursing faculty have the potential to extend their influence to students in other health care professionals and shape the future of interprofessional practice.

References

Allen P. Preparing nurses for tomorrow's healthcare system. *American Nurse Today.* 2013;8(5):46–50.

Brady D, Welborn-Brown P, Smith D, et al. Staying afloat: surviving curriculum change. *Nurse Educ.* 2008;33(5):198–201.

Brandon AF, All AC. Constructivism theory analysis and application to curricula. *Nurs Educ Perspect.* 2010;31(2):89–92.

Deane W, Asselin M. Transitioning to concept-based teaching: a discussion of strategies and the use of Bridges change model. *J Nurs Educ Pract.* 2015;5(10):52–58.

Decker K, Hensel D, Kuhn T, Priest C. Innovative implementation of social determinants of health in a new concept-based curriculum. *Nurse Educ.* 2017;42(3):115–116.

Duncan K, Schulz PS. Impact of change to a concept-based baccalaureate nursing curriculum on student and program outcomes. *J Nurs Educ.* 2015;54(3):S16–S20.

Erickson HL, Lanning LA. *Transitioning to Concept-based Curriculum and Instruction.* Thousand Oaks, CA: Corwin Publishing; 2014.

Fromer R. Theory integrative process/outcome evaluation of a concept-based curriculum. *Nurs Educ Perspect.* 2017;38(5):267–269.

Getha-Eby TJ, Beery T, O'Brien B, Xu Y. Student learning outcomes in response to concept-based teaching. *J Nurs Educ.* 2015;54(4):193–200.

Giddens J, Brady D. Rescuing nursing education from content saturation: the case for a concept-based curriculum. *J Nurs Educ.* 2007;46:65–69.

Giddens J, Morton N. Report card: An evaluation of a concept-based curriculum. *Nurs Educ Perspect.* 2010;31(6):372–377.

Giddens J, Brady D, Brown P, Wright M, Smith D, Harris J. A new curriculum for a new era of nursing education. *Nurs Educ Perspect.* 2008;29(4):200–204.

Giddens J, Wright M, Gray I. Selecting concepts for a concept-based curriculum: application of a benchmark approach. *J Nurs Educ.* 2012;51(9):511–519.

Giddens J. Underestimated challenges adopting the conceptual approach. *J Nurs Educ.* 2016;55(4):187–188.

Goodman T. Nursing education moves to a concept-based curriculum. *Association of periOperative Registered Nurses Connections.* 2014;99(6):C7–C8.

Gooder V, Cantwell S. Student experiences with a newly developed concept-based curriculum. *Teach Learn Nurs*. 2017;12(2):142–147.

Hardin PK, Richardson SJ. Teaching the concept curricula: theory and method. *J Nurs Educ*. 2012;51(3): 155–159.

Harrison S, Gibbons C. Nursing student perceptions of concept maps: from theory to practice. *Nurs Educ Perspect*. 2013;34(6):395–399.

Heims ML, Boyd ST. Concept-based learning activities in clinical nursing education. *Nurs Educ Perspect*. 1990;29(6):249–254.

Hensel D. Using Q methodology to assess learning outcomes following the implementation of a concept-based curriculum. *Nurse Educ*. 2017;42(5):250–254.

Hendricks S, Wangerin V. Concept-based curriculum: changing attitudes and overcoming barriers. *Nurse Educ*. 2017;42(3):138–142.

Higgins B, Reid H. Enhancing conceptual teaching/learning in a concept-based curriculum. *Teach Learn Nurs*. 2016;12:95–102.

Hollinshead J, Stirling L. A conceptual curriculum framework designed to ensure quality student health visitor training in practice. *Community Pract*. 2014;87(7):22–25.

Institute of Medicine. *Health Professions Education: A Bridge to Quality*. Washington DC: National Academy Press; 2003.

Interprofessional Education Collaborative. *Core Competencies for Interprofessional Practice: 2016 Update*. Washington DC: Interprofessional Education Collaborative; 2016.

Kantor SA. Pedagogical change in nursing education: one instructor's experience. *J Nurs Educ*. 2010;49(7): 414–417.

Laasater K, Nielsen A. The influence on concept-based learning activities on students' clinical judgement development. *J Nurs Educ*. 2009;48(8):441–446.

Lanz A, Davis RG. Pharmacology goes concept-based: course design, implementation, and evaluation. *Nurs Educ Perspect*. 2017;38(5):279–280.

Laverentz DM, Kumm S. Concept evaluation using the PDSA cycle for continuous quality improvement. *Nurs Educ Perspect*. 2017;38(5):288–290.

Lee-Hsieh J, Kao C, Kuo C, Tseng H. Clinical nursing competence of RN-BSN students in a nursing concept-based curriculum in taiwan. *J Nurs Educ*. 2003;42(12):536–545.

Lewis L. Outcomes of a concept-based curriculum. *Teach Learn Nurs*. 2014;9(2):75–79.

McGrath B. The development of a concept-based learning approach as part of an integrative nursing curriculum. *Whitireia Nursing and Health Journal*. 2015;22:11–17.

Mood LC, Neunzert C, Tadesse R. Centering the concept of transitional care: a teaching-learning innovation. *J Nurs Educ*. 2014;53(5):287–290.

Murray S, Laurent K, Gontarz J. Evaluation of a concept-based curriculum: a tool and process. *Teach Learn Nurs*. 2015;10:169–175.

Nelson-Brantley H, Laverentz DM. Leaderless organization: active learning strategy in a concept-based curriculum. *J Nurs Educ*. 2014;53(8):484.

Nielsen A. Concept-based learning activities using the clinical judgement model as a foundation for clinical learning. *J Nurs Educ*. 2009;48(6):350–354.

Nielsen A, Noone J, Voss H, Mathews LR. Preparing students for the future: an innovative approach to clinical education. *Nurs Educ Pract*. 2013;13:301–309.

Nielsen A. Concept-based learning in clinical experiences: bringing theory to clinical education for deep learning. *J Nurs Educ*. 2016;55(7):365–371.

Patterson LD, Crager JM, Farmer A, Epps CD, Schuessler JB. A strategy to ensure faculty engagement when assessing a concept-based curriculum. *J Nurs Educ*. 2016;55(8):467–470.

Popoola M. Popoola Holistic Praxis Model—a framework for curriculum development. *West Afr J Nurs*. 2012;23(2):43–56.

Senita J. The use of concept maps to evaluate critical thinking in the clinical setting. *Teach Learn Nurs*. 2008;3(1):6–10.

Taylor L, Littleton-Keamey M. Concept mapping: a distinctive educational approach to foster critical thinking. *Nurse Educ*. 2011;36(2):84–88.

Trossman SA. Change in the air: nurses discuss value of a concept-based approach to education. *Am Nurse*. 2015. http://www.theamericannurse.org/2015/08/31/a-change-in-the-air/.

APPENDIX A

Clinical Activities Focusing on Concepts

Linda Caputi

The activities in this Appendix are examples of learning that focus students' perceptual awareness on the study of concepts in the clinical setting. The focused clinical learning activities provide an in-depth study of a concept. The students completing the assignment present their work in post-conference and/or submit their work as part of required assignments for the clinical course. All students learn from that work and are expected to use that learning in the care of patients in a variety of health care settings throughout the nursing program. The thinking required to complete the assignment is of equal importance to the study of the concept.

Focused Clinical Learning Activity: Concept—Evidence

Evidence-Based Practice Guidelines

The purpose of this assignment is to learn about practice guidelines. The National Guidelines Clearinghouse is a public resource for evidence-based practice guidelines. Visit the National Guidelines Clearinghouse website (www.guidelines.gov) and find one evidence-based practice guideline that applies to a patient you are caring for. Also find and review one other source for evidence-based nursing care that can be applied to your patient. Write a summary based on the following:

1. Provide a brief explanation of the care you are providing.
2. What guidelines did you investigate?
3. In what way were the medical orders and the care provided by members of the health care team consistent with the guidelines? In what way were these different?
4. Did you change your approach to care after reading these guidelines? If so, how? If not, why not?

Focused Clinical Learning Activity: Concept—Patient Education

Discharge Teaching Incorporating the Concepts of *Development* and *Culture*

The purpose of this assignment is to prepare discharge instructions and determine teaching needs of your patient. Consider how the patient's age and developmental level (Concept of Development) and culture (Concept of Culture) will affect your teaching. Identify who you will teach, their literacy level, and their knowledge base related to the information you will be teaching. Use the following questions to focus your teaching planning.

Guiding questions:

1. Is patient/family ready to learn?
2. What learning outcomes must occur before the patient/family can be discharged?
3. What are the patient's/family's perceived learning needs?
4. Are there barriers to learning (language, literacy, stress, physical distractions)?
5. How does the patient/family wish to have information presented (verbal, written, chart/diagram)?
6. How will you evaluate the learning outcomes?

Focused Clinical Learning Activity: Concept—Health Care Organizations

Analyzing the Clinical Microsystem

For this learning activity, go to the Microsystem Academy website http://www.clinicalmicrosystem.org/knowledge-center/workbooks and retrieve the document: *Inpatient Workbook.* While you are on the clinical unit, complete the two following tools found in this workbook:

- Inpatient Unit Profile (on page 6)
- Inpatient Unit Unplanned Activity Tracking Card (on page 16)

Answer the following questions:

1. What did you learn about an inpatient unit that you were not aware of?
2. What aspects of the clinical microsystem did you recognize that might lead to nurses making errors?
3. What changes can be made on the unit to prevent errors?

Concept of Health Care Quality

Activity: Nursing-Sensitive Indicators/Quality Improvement Measures

1. What nursing-sensitive indicators and quality improvement projects are in use on the unit?
2. What nursing-sensitive indicators and quality measures apply to your patient?
3. How are the nursing-sensitive quality indicators measured?
4. What screening tools are used?
5. What gaps are present in patient care and how will you apply the nursing-sensitive indicators and quality improvement projects to improve patient care?

Concept of Technology and Informatics

Activity: Analyzing Technology

Type of technology (List all technology used: computer charting, fetal monitors, IV pumps, pulse oximeters, etc.)	How the technology is used	Who accesses the technology	How does the technology contribute to safe, quality care?

Describe how you used the technology.	Discuss your application of the technology to document patient care.

Example of a Teaching Strategy: Compare and Contrast Patients With an Infection

Factors to Consider	Patient 1	Patient 2	Patient 3
Type of infection/pathophysiology			
Preexisting conditions			
Medications prescribed			
Age-related considerations			
Attributes of the concept of *Infection* most affecting the patient			
Interrelated concepts			
Concepts to Consider	**Patient 1**	**Patient 2**	**Patient 3**
Care Coordination			
Patient Education			
Developmental Level			
Health Care Environment			
Health Promotion			
Ethics			
Add other concepts important to these patients.			

Discussion and Reflection Questions for the Concept of Collaboration in the Home Setting

- Based on the definition of "collaborate," how would you apply collaboration in the home health setting?
- Who are the team members (including the patient and the patient's support persons) with whom you will collaborate?
- Describe a situation in which you experienced effective or successful collaboration with others when working in the home setting. Why was the collaboration effective or successful?
- Describe a situation in which you experienced ineffective or unsuccessful collaboration with others when working in the home setting. Why was it unsuccessful?

Example of a FCLA for Culture

Cultural Assessment as it Pertains to Health Preferences

Learning Activity: Conduct a cultural assessment on four individuals from racial, ethnic, and cultural backgrounds different from your own. For each person, include their age and the cultural group(s) with which they identify, and use the information in the box below to base your conversation.

Data to Include as Part of a Cultural Assessment

Origins and Family

- Where born—if in other country, length of time living in this country and what brought them here.
- Description of the family and family members
- How decisions are made in family
- Cultural practices shared by family

Daily Practices

- Spiritual beliefs and religious practices
- Dietary preferences, practices, forbidden foods
- Beliefs regarding foods that pertain to health and illness
- Special rituals
- Practices or routines to maintain or improve health

Communication

- Language spoken at home; skill in reading, writing, speaking in English
- Preferred methods to communicate
- Ways respect is shown, particularly when communicating
- Preferences, practices regarding eye contact, personal space, touch

Personal Beliefs about Health and Illness

- Perception of one's control over health
- Meaning of illness; perception of illness severity
- Expectations and preferences regarding treatment practices
- Concerns or fears regarding health care; practices that violate beliefs (taboos)

Adapted from: Caplan. Culture. In: Giddens J, ed. *Concepts for Nursing Practice.* 2nd ed. St. Louis, MO: Elsevier; 2017.

Assignment: Write up your findings for each of the four individuals you interviewed. Then address the following questions: 1) What similarities and differences do you notice in the findings? 2) Was there anything that surprised you? 3) How did this activity broaden your understanding of culture? 4) How will you apply what was learned in future patient interactions?

Preparing a Concept for Concept-Based Teaching: Explanation and Template

Beth Rodgers

Concept-based teaching requires a change in the traditional teaching model. To be effective at concept-based teaching, it is essential to be clear about the concepts that are being taught. Consistency in preparation and approach can be helpful to students as they learn the concepts presented in the curriculum. Thorough preparation with regard to phenomena, concepts, language, related concepts, contexts, and exemplars are critical to the success of teaching concepts.

The steps that are described in this section can be used to identify phenomena and associated concepts, to ensure the best language and terminology are used, and to help organize ideas for presenting the concept to students. Discussed below is a listing of the components necessary for teaching related to a concept and discussion of each element.

At the end of this material, there is a template that can be used for additional concept clarification. The template can be used along with the components of concept presentation that were addressed in Chapter 6. Once the concept is defined clearly, presentation should include assessment, populations and risk factors, and clinical management, as well as physiological processes, theoretical links, and other aspects that are appropriate for students to grasp the concept and its application.

Step1: What Is the Phenomenon?

A phenomenon is an experience as it is perceived by the person having the experience, and a short narrative about the phenomenon can be an excellent starting point. Concepts are used to organize experience, and the experiences that are organized are based on phenomena. For example, the phenomenon of interest for a class session may be how the body regulates temperature or the amount of heat in the body. This phenomenon appears in situations of merely being alive, as a certain temperature or degree of heat is essential for human life. There is more heat when there are inflammatory or infectious processes occurring (and other examples), and heat is reduced when blood vessels dilate to dissipate heat such as in cases of shock. Exposure to cold external temperatures can cause the body to lose heat and make adjustments to maintain the temperature necessary for survival of the brain and organs. This phenomenon is associated with a number of concepts, one of which is *Heat*. If the focus is on how heat is balanced, then the concept might be *Thermoregulation*. If the focus is only on insufficient heat, the concept could be *Hypothermia*.

Do not identify the concept at this point; keep the focus on the situation that is of interest. Keep the emphasis on what is happening, looking at the situation as if it were something new. Once you are certain of the situation or experience of interest, then begin to think about what concepts might apply and the appropriate words to use. It is common to approach a situation with a number of labels in mind, and then the words can drive the observation. In this activity, it is important that the concepts and language emerge from the situation rather than being applied to it to avoid a mismatch of concepts and phenomenon. Step 3 will help with the application of language to the phenomenon.

Step 2: Where Is the Phenomenon Found?

This discussion can be included with the description, above, if that is easier. In some cases, discussion of the situation or cases in which the phenomenon is encountered can be illuminating. For example, is heat associated only with environmental exposure or can it be found in other contexts? Continuing with the example of *Thermoregulation*, this phenomenon is found in all cases of animal life. In regard to nursing, the phenomenon of thermoregulation can be found in all situations that involve human beings. It is not specific to age, setting, wellness or illness orientation, or other factors. It is inherent in working with humans in any manner. Encourage students to think outside of the typical circumstances as a way to reinforce the understanding of the concept.

Step 3: What Is the Concept and Appropriate Terminology?

After completing the steps above, the appropriate concepts will come into focus for the teaching-learning experience. Keep in mind that the concept is not the same as the word! Identification of the concept needs to involve selection of the appropriate word. Concepts can be expressed using different terminology that sometimes, but not always, conveys the same characteristics. Is there a difference in *Temperature Regulation* and *Thermoregulation*? What is the "best" terminology to use as the focus? Acknowledging other terminology that conveys the same concept can help students avoid confusion and expand their ability to communicate with others. The "best" terminology most likely is that used by nurses in their professional context and that reflects current evidence.

Step 4: What Other Concepts Are Similar or Related?

No concept exists in a vacuum. A concept is part of a complex network of related ideas, connected in some way, due to similarity, difference, or interdependence. *Thermoregulation*, for example, is related to *Metabolism, Circulation,* and a variety of other concepts. Identifying these connections can help to structure the presentation of a concept to students so they do not view concepts and related phenomena in isolation. In some cases, discussion of similar concepts is essential to clarifying the primary concept of interest. *Grief* and *Bereavement*, for example, sometimes are discussed as interchangeable, yet recognizing the difference in these two concepts is critical to understanding the experience of loss and the associated response. *Sleepiness* and *Fatigue* can be confused easily, yet failure to differentiate which concept is appropriate in a particular situation can result in missed problem identification and ineffective treatment plans.

Step 5: What Are the Key Components (Attributes) of the Concept?

Having selected the concept and the appropriate terminology to express it, the critical process of identifying the key components of the concept can begin. The purpose here is to identify the essential aspects of the concept, specifically the attributes of the concept. This can be done by selecting exemplary cases to analyze, reviewing current and quality literature to analyze discussions of the concept, etc. See Chapter 3, *Development of Concepts for Concept-Based Teaching*, for more information about components (attributes) of concepts.

Step 6: What Is the Context for an Instance of the Concept?

Context includes a description of the general situation in which an example of the concept is appropriate. In the case of *Thermoregulation*, contexts include infection, exposure, exercise, anything that causes vascular change, certain neurologic conditions, and maintenance of basal metabolism. The context similarly includes a temporal element, including precipitating events and outcomes. Precipitating events sometimes are part of the context (such as exposure) but also may include antecedents such as medications that cause vasodilation or an increase in activity level. Consequences, or outcomes, of thermoregulation include, if the concept is executed successfully, maintenance of an optimal body temperature. Consequences, or outcomes, may also include results of ineffective regulation such as hypo- or hyperthermia. The thermoregulatory mechanism itself involves physiological responses such as change in the peripheral vascular system, sweating, and if those are successful, optimal temperature is maintained in the body. This question of context involves a number of facets that are critical to an understanding of the concept.

Step 7: Present Examples

Examples may be developed based on the clinical experience of the instructor, situations the students see in their clinical experience, examples found in the literature, or case studies based on a multitude of sources. Examples should not be thought of as the "model cases," as seen commonly in many approaches to concept analysis. It is important that students be confronted with the wide range of variation in a concept, not merely the ideal or model cases. They will see concepts on a dynamic continuum; encourage students to keep an open mind as knowledge changes and concepts change with that new knowledge. Examples help students learn to apply the concept effectively, but should not be construed or presented in a manner that could place limits on conceptual understanding. The examples that are most appropriate in the teaching-learning situation will vary based on the learning experience and the focus on the conceptual teaching.

Template for Concept Clarification

1. What is the phenomenon?
2. Where is the phenomenon found?
3. What is the concept?
   A. Identify the best term or label for the concept that relates to the phenomenon.
   B. What other terms are used to express the concept? (same idea/concept, but alternate terms)
4. What other concepts are similar or related? Describe differences and similarities.
5. What are the key components (attributes) of the concept?
6. What are common contexts for the concept?
   A. The concept is likely to apply in what situations?
   B. What are precipitating factors or events?
   C. What are outcomes or results?
7. Develop or describe examples. Consider the range of variation and not just ideal examples.

INDEX

Note: Page numbers followed by "f" indicate figures, "t" indicate tables and "b" indicate boxes.

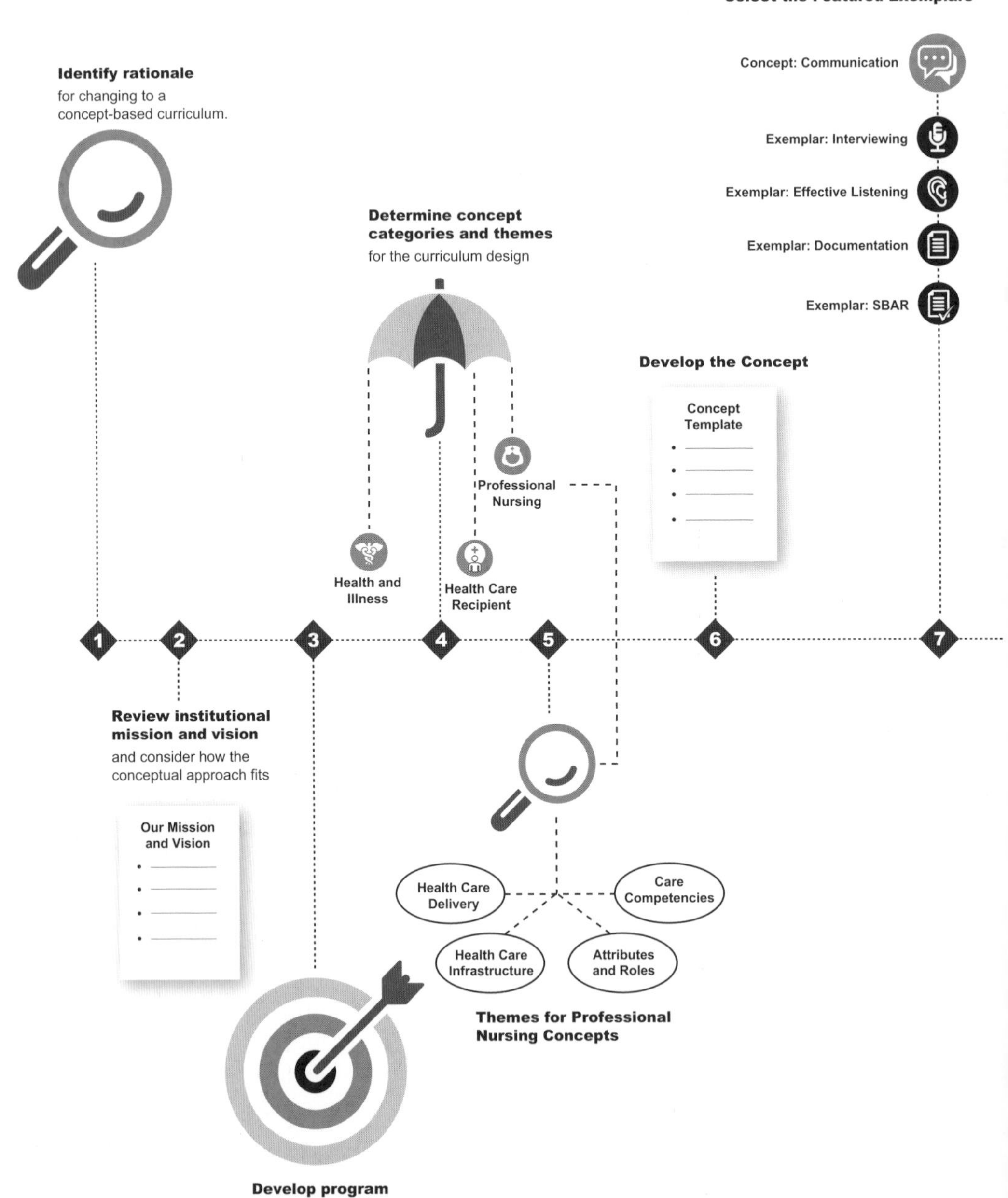
Select the Featured Exemplars
Concept: Communication
Exemplar: Interviewing
Exemplar: Effective Listening
Exemplar: Documentation
Exemplar: SBAR
Identify rationale
for changing to a concept-based curriculum.
Determine concept categories and themes
for the curriculum design
Professional Nursing
Health and Illness
Health Care Recipient
Develop the Concept
Concept Template
1
2
3
4
5
6
7
Review institutional mission and vision
and consider how the conceptual approach fits
Our Mission and Vision
Health Care Delivery
Care Competencies
Health Care Infrastructure
Attributes and Roles
Themes for Professional Nursing Concepts
Develop program outcomes and/or competencies